To Sleep

A flock of sheep that leisurely pass by
One after one; the sound of rain, and bees
Murmuring; the fall of rivers, wind and seas,
Smooth fields, white sheets of water and pure sky;
I've thought of all by turns, and still I lie
Sleepless; and soon the small birds' melodies
I must hear, first utter'd from my orchard trees,
And the first Cuckoo's melancholy cry.
Even thus last night, and two nights more, I lie,
And could not coin thee, Sleep! by any stealth:
So do not let me wear to-night away.
Without thee what is all the morning's wealth?
Come, blessed barrier betwixt day and day,
Dear mother of fresh thoughts and joyous health.

William Wordsworth

the Sleep Book

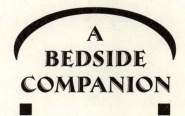

A BEDSIDE COMPANION

Jody Grant–Gray

To my husband, Don, for his patience during my years of sleeplessness. And our son, Coleman, whose years of sleeplessness have taught me patience.

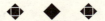

The material contained herein is for information only, and is not designed to replace medical diagnosis or treatment. See a trained medical professional before taking any medicaton, if your sleeplessness is ongoing, or if your sleeplessness gives any indication of a more general health problem.

Copyright © 2000, Jody Grant-Gray.

All rights reserved. No part of this book may be reproduced, except for short excerpts used in reviews, without the written permission of the publisher. For information, contact:

Aero U.S.
P.O. Box # 7623
Santa Monica, CA. 90406-7623
www.aerous.com

Library of Congress Card Number: 00-100277

ISBN: 0-9670351-0-4 Health/Fitness

Printed in Canada

Contents

A Practical Consideration of Sleep and Sleeplessness, A to Z
pages 7–215

Index
pages 216–221

Acknowledgments
page 222

Note:

Words **bold** in text indicate chapter
headings bearing that title.

Ability

I have not slept a wink.
Alexander Pope
Imitations of Horace, 1738.

Some people just have the ability to sleep.

And you don't. At least, that is what you may be thinking as you begin to explore this book.

Perhaps you are hopeful. You should be; the success rate for correcting problem sleep is remarkably high. Or you may feel frustrated. Understandably; most people trying to improve their sleep have had to make their way with little or no direction. In all likelihood, you feel a little of both, along with myriad other emotions surrounding those hours from dusk to dawn.

No small art it is to sleep!
It is necessary for that purpose
to keep awake all day.
Friedrich Nietzche
Thus Spake Zarathustra, 1892.

You may be one of those despairing of *ever* having sound, satisfying sleep on a regular basis, or questioning your competence in what so many others consider a simple task. Let me reassure you. *You have the ability to sleep*. Documented cases of people physically unable to sleep are exceedingly rare.

In beginning this book, you are already demonstrating one quality, desire, that will help determine your future success. You should consider it, then, not a question of *if* you will fall asleep, as much as *when*, and *how well*. This book can help you attain a restful, quality sleep sooner than you may have ever thought possible.

In the meantime, learn about sleep, about yourself, and how to rest easy... for life! You have the ability to sleep. And you will sleep. It's that simple.

Achievement

With the ever-increasing attention given the subject, it may sometimes seem that you must be an expert on sleep in order to even achieve it. You don't. You don't have to explain the process, or be able to teach others. You just need to find out *what works for you*.

The **cause** of your troubled sleep may seem elusive, especially at first. It could be a bad habit, or less than ideal physical conditions. It may be a health problem that can only be solved with medical intervention. It might be stress, or frustration, that keeps you staring at the ceiling night after night. Most likely, it is a combination of several factors. And, like any puzzle, you must consider your current situation to discover which pieces are needed for the solution, and where they will fit.

Don't expect that some generic answer exists that will fix everything; instead assume that each situation, *your* situation, requires unique measures. Learn about sleep. Talk to your doctor. Exercise patience: even after determining the cause of your sleeplessness, relief may not be immediately forthcoming. Experiment with different techniques to find those most effective. Recognize that what was successful for a group of laboratory subjects may not necessarily produce results for *you*.

Think of sleep as a subjective question, in which there is no *correct* answer. You may be a better sleeper if you change the bed clothes nightly. You may only achieve a good night's rest in the comfort of familiar surroundings. You may need to sleep with the light on, the window open, or the covers pulled up over your head. What *most* people do matters little, if it does not help *you* to sleep.

Rest easy, knowing that you are beginning a great journey, on your way to a wonderful discovery—you. What makes you sleep. What keeps you from it. With effort, practice, and desire, you can become an accomplished sleeper. A good night's sleep is a simple yet great satisfaction, and you will have yourself to thank.

> *"Some are born with the knowledge...some know by study; and some acquire the knowledge after a painful feeling of their ignorance...But the achievement being made, it comes to the same thing."*
>
> Confucius
> *The Doctrine of the Mean*, 500 B.C.

Anticipation

> So much did we feel ourselves to be already at home, in anticipation, that...many on board, to whom this was the first voyage, could scarcely sleep.
>
> Richard Henry Dana
> *Two Years Before the Mast*, 1840.

Tomorrow is your big day. It could be your graduation or wedding, the vacation you're beginning, or the surgery you're dreading. It may be your first date with someone new, or the feared breakup lunch; your child's first day at kindergarten, or their going away to college. You may feel every upcoming day is a big day; an admirable attitude. But how are you supposed to sleep *tonight*?

At the risk of sounding simplistic: the best you can. You might try going to bed a little earlier than usual if you anticipate tossing and turning, suffering a delayed onset sleep. Or stick to your normal routine if a change will cause even more anxiety. This is a situation where you can expect to have some trouble sleeping.

It's *temporary*, so don't berate yourself over your inability to sleep; instead take comfort in the extenuating nature of the circumstances, and the fact that you will still realize some benefits from this less than perfect 'night before'.

And above all, keep things in perspective: it *is* your big day tomorrow, so rejoice! It means you are alive, and awake (literally and figuratively) to all the possibilities the day offers.

Now, get some sleep (as much as possible), so you don't greet this day with dark circles under your eyes!

> *I had but a broken sleep the night before, in anticipation of the pleasure of a whole day with Em'ly.*
>
> Charles Dickens
> *David Copperfield*, 1850.

Breathe

> *No life that breathes with human breath*
> *Has ever truly longed for death.*
> Lord Alfred Tennyson
> *The Two Voices*, 1832.

We manage it unconsciously and continuously, while awake and while asleep; collecting and distributing, through the process of respiration, the oxygen needed by our bodies. And unless you are one of those prone to talking or walking about, automatic responses like breathing become the foremost concern of our physical bodies while sleeping.

To consider it strictly as an unconscious action, however, is to overlook a great deal of what breathing has to offer. For instance, the famous illusionist Harry Houdini considered his technique for breath control, developed through years of training, to be the foundation of his celebrated escape acts. Hypnosis, especially self-hypnosis, emphasizes breathing as a conduit to the suggestible, hypnotic state. And nearly all types of meditation have controlled, conscious breathing at their centers.

Conscious breathing can help you listen to your physical self; it is communication without the mental "chatter" of language, which can often overwhelm. In conscious breathing, you are always in complete control.

For the troubled sleeper, even some basic breathing techniques can yield benefits, both for your sleep and your overall health.

While you're reading now, try this: breathe in, deeply yet not too quickly. Hold it for just a moment, then release, a bit slower than it took to bring the breath in, but equally deeply. With that simple act you have taken an important step toward relaxation, and by extension, improved sleep: you have shifted your emphasis on breathing from the exclusively physical (unconscious) to the mental (conscious) state.

Try it again, with a few refinements:

This time, be aware of the physical movements and changes in your body when you inhale. Feel your chest rise, and expand; your stomach swell slightly; your shoulders (especially if you are sitting, rather than reclining) lift to accommodate the intake of air. Consider the size of the breath you take: not to capacity, which would cause discomfort, but enough to fill the lungs generously.

The pause between your inhale and exhale is not really a "hold"; think of it more as that point a ball eventually reaches when thrown up into the air: between rising and falling, when gravity is no longer being overcome, yet has not begun to exert its pull.

As you exhale, be aware of how those muscles involved in the process feel: the response is not relief as much as a feeling of rejuvenation, of energizing relaxation.

From the individual breath, look to the *pattern* of your breathing. Regular, unhurried, like the shore lap of a calm sea, each breath is a unique entity unto itself, but exists only as part of a seamless continuum. Like a mark made on the edge of a slowly rotating wheel, each breath is equal parts rising and falling, introduction and conclusion; and another breath is already begun even at the moment the last has ended.

We could hear her gentle breathing as she slept;
gradually it became quieter and calmer, and on
her countenance beamed happiness and peace.
Hans Christian Andersen
Fairy Tales, 1835-72.

With each breath you relax further, going deeper and deeper into a placid calm. Don't think of your breathing as the direct *cause* of your increasing relaxation, but a means of *transportation*; like the passing signs on a highway, each breath means you are further along.

Every night you have the opportunity to take this relaxing, yet rejuvenating, journey. The more often you travel the route, the shorter and more familiar it becomes. With practice, controlled, conscious breathing will announce to your mind and body not just that the trip has begun, but that the destination is already in sight.

"You might just as well say," added the
Dormouse, which seemed to be talking in its
sleep, "that 'I breathe when I sleep' is the same
thing as 'I sleep when I breathe'!"
"It is the same thing with you," said the Hatter,
and here the conversation dropped, and the
party sat silent for a minute...

Bruxism

"In my youth," said his father, "I took to the
law, and argued each case with my wife; and
the muscular strength, which it gave to my jaw,
has lasted the rest of my life."
Lewis Carroll
Alice's Adventures in Wonderland, 1865.

Bruxism is a name given that condition more commonly known as *grinding your teeth*. It occurs, in one form or another, in millions of people. For a great many,

12

this habitual clenching of the jaw and/or grinding of the teeth occurs while in bed, sleeping.

Or not sleeping; since the sound of grinding is often loud enough to awaken both the sleeper and their bed partner.

Besides premature wear to the teeth, bruxism can cause a number of different gum problems, severe damage to the joints of the jaw (often grouped under the heading *temporomandibular joint disorders,* or *TMJ*), and even adversely affect your looks— the overdevelopment of the *masseter* muscles can contribute to a "chipmunk cheeks" appearance. In extreme cases, when it is time to wake up, you may not even be able to open your mouth!

Grinding your teeth while sleeping could be just a bad habit, or it can have at it roots psychological causes, including increased stress or anxiety. Even if it doesn't awaken you, it can adversely affect the quality of your sleep, as well as your overall health. Unfortunately, unless it is witnessed by someone other than the sleeper, it can be difficult to diagnose. A dentist may detect unusual wear to the teeth, but headaches, ear aches, and a stiff or sore neck may be symptoms of bruxism, as well.

Once diagnosed by your dentist or specialist, treatment can take several forms. Muscle relaxants and anti-depressants may be prescribed, with all the problems of adverse reactions and dependencies that accompany them. If the grinding is from habit, a mouthguard-like *splint,* or *night guard,* can be particularly effective; so much so that once the behavior is modified, you may find you don't always need to wear it.

If the cause of the clenching and grinding is stress, and it quite often is, the pre-sleep or relaxation techniques found in this book and others may prove helpful. Programs of *self-hypnosis* therapy may also be prescribed by your health professional. While results of such programs *can* be dramatic, you should be aware:

the more ingrained the stress and the underlying behavior that fosters it, the more difficult it can be to correct; and also, the effectiveness of self-hypnosis programs are contingent on the continuing suggestibility of the subject (you), so *stick with them*.

If you suspect you are grinding or clenching your teeth, see your dentist; both for recommendations and to check for damage (and don't forget to floss regularly to avoid that nasty lecture!). Your sleep, and your health, may depend on it.

En boca cerrada no entran moscas.
(The closed mouth swallows no flies.)
Spanish Proverb

Busy

Nowher so bisy a man as he ther nas,
And yet he seemed bisier than he was.
Geoffrey Chaucer,
The Canterbury Tales, 1387

There aren't enough hours in the day to finish your work, run all your errands, meet all your obligations. But you try.

In the evening, as tired as you are, you rouse yourself to work on your screenplay, fold your laundry, or write your bills before bed. You still have to check your e-mail and respond to those most important, and in the background you catch a half hour of the game or movie you so optimistically taped, just to make that effort worthwhile. Before you know it, it's that time: so off to bed you go, to start over for the next day.

There is a time for many words,
and there is also a time
for sleep.
Homer

14

But once in your bed, you can't relax. Your mind is buzzing, racing, coming up with still more unfinished or hitherto forgotten tasks. It is even (gasp) organizing them into *to-do lists*. Your body is certainly tired enough, but where is the peace, the solitude, the quiet that so many times throughout the day you found yourself longing for? If you cannot find it there, in the darkness of your room, then you need to make some changes.

Too busy with the crowded hour,
to fear to live or die.
Ralph Waldo Emerson

Don't make work while at rest. Don't make to-do lists in bed, even (especially?) if you have a lot on your mind. Take care of this kind of mental activity during the day, and preferably well before bedtime. If it does have to happen late into the night, use it as a pre-sleep **ritual** on the order of brushing your teeth. Give yourself a half hour to sit quietly, and compose all your thoughts. Write them down, if you must, but once you've entered them into your palm PC, or locked them in your briefcase, forget about them until morning.

For those that have particular difficulty letting go of tasks, try this: make it a point to assign a *specific time* each night for such mental activities. Consider your various projects, your unfinished business, but only for this designated time, then quit for the night; no matter how tempting it is to go back and take on "just one more thing".

You may well be the type of person who has to keep a dozen balls in the air at once. Shortchanging yourself on sleep, though, will only make the juggling harder.

O! That man
may know the end
of this day's business,
ere it come.
William Shakespeare
Julius Caesar, 1599.

15

Casbah

*He knew well what he wanted, and he sent away
the women and maidens. When that was done,
the king himself locked the door, and shot two
strong bolts before it. He hid the light quickly
behind the bed curtain, and the struggle that
had to come began, between stark Siegfried and
the beautiful maiden...*

Anon.
The Nibelungenlied, c.1200.

For privacy, romance, intimacy and adventure, invest in a curtained bed. With a tug of the drapes you can shut out the rest of the world, and be in your own little cocoon. Even as a three year old, my son would pull the bed covers over his head to sleep, though the room was dark and quiet. Do we ever outgrow the womb-like appeal of private sleep?

My husband thinks they're feminine. For the testosterone driven, then, go native: the classic mosquito netting (after all, Papa Hemingway, John Huston, and Clark Gable all slept under it) can achieve the same result in a decidedly more manly fashion.

Turn your bedroom into the casbah; create the night of a thousand veils. Shut out the world and seduce, reproduce, and fall into luscious and sensuous sleep, night after night. Sleep alone? Wherever you are becomes a world of luxury and privacy, an environment once the realm of kings and queens. An uncommon world for an uncommon sleep.

*To create a public scandal
is what's wicked;
to sin in private is not a sin.*
Moliere
Tartuffe, 1664.

■ ⊞ ■

Catch up

...I do not remember now what the resting consisted of, for when we got back to Naples we had not slept for forty-eight hours. We were just about to go to bed early in the evening, and catch up on some of the sleep we had lost, when we heard of this Vesuvius expedition...

Mark Twain
The Innocents Abroad, 1869.

You *can* "catch up" on your sleep. A few nights without it will not be the end of you, nor lead to disaster. There are no lasting effects to a couple of consecutive nights with little or no sleep (excepting, of course, if those nights occur in Las Vegas or Atlantic City). Laboratory controlled deprivation experiments have demonstrated that as little as eight hours of sleep can restore a person after several days without it.

The point here is this: you do not have to feel you've fallen into a downward spiral after a couple of rough nights; even months of substandard sleep can be overcome with just a few nights of **quality** sleep. Unlike most other situations in life, a lot of bad *can* be undone with a little good, and the sleep problems that may have been troubling you for years can be resolved in significantly less time than you may realize.

Do not see your situation as hopeless, even though to this point you may have had little success; instead feel confident that quality sleep, when it does come, will bring renewal. Don't create a situation where the pressure to succeed is contributing to failure: like a hectic vacation that leaves you more frazzled than rested, working hard at relaxation (a critical component of sleep) can produce the opposite effect.

Tonight's wakefulness does not mean the end of your good health. When you eventually catch up on your sleep (and you will), appreciate how much better you feel. In the meantime, rest easy knowing that, if not tonight, or even this week, your body will forgive your sleeplessness and eventually restore you to your full potential.

Causes

*There is occasions
and causes
why and wherefore
in all things.*
William Shakespeare
King Henry the Fifth, 1600.

Western medicine is predicated a great deal on the concept: *find the cause to find the cure*. The study of sleep and sleep disorders has, for the most part, proven this axiom. While there are almost countless reasons for problem sleep, the success rate for getting people to sleep, once they have been diagnosed, is remarkably high.

The first step in improving your sleep, then, is to determine *why* you are not sleeping. The cause (unfortunately) could be any number of things, alone or in combination. Often you are caught up in a vicious cycle. Because you are not sleeping well, you are more vulnerable in your waking hours. Because you are more vulnerable, you feel you are not coping well, that your actions are compromised. At night, when you should be sleeping, you find yourself going over your day, wondering if you could have handled things better. Before you know it, your night has passed without enough sleep; you're left facing another day of misguided decisions, and sensitivity to otherwise minor emotional disturbances.

I mention this here because it is estimated that fully *one half* of all sleep problems have a psychological basis. You may be under a great deal of pressure at work, or in your home life. Stress reduction techniques can help you to deal with this increased tension. While eliminating the cause of the stress is most effective, it is not always possible (to say the least); but without reducing either its cause, or your response to it, your sleep will be compromised.

> *What hath night*
> *to do with sleep?*
> John Milton
> *Comus*, 1634.

The reason for your sleeplessness may be primarily physical. It could be a sleep related condition like *sleep apnea* which involves sudden stoppages of breath throughout the night, or periodic limb movements (*nocturnal myoclonus*), that has you waking up repeatedly. It could be a more general health problem that only manifests itself while you are sleeping, like leg cramps, or heartburn. It could be a problem like dehydration, or a vitamin or mineral deficiency, that develops over the course of the day but culminates at that time so critical to your body's repair and rejuvenation.

The physical problem may not even be your own, but your bedmate's: *their* snoring, grinding their teeth (**bruxism**), or walking or talking in their sleep, could be what's keeping *you* awake.

The reason could be merely a question of physical **comfort**: you could just be too hot or cold, or sleeping on too hard, too soft, or too lumpy a mattress.

In sleeplessness, finding the cause *can* help you find the **cure**. It may take hard work and perseverance. It may take some creativity. It may take medical intervention. It will probably take some time. But what have you got to lose? Stop losing sleep over losing sleep. Get aggressive about figuring out the cause (either by yourself or with assis-

19

tance), and determine the best solution(s) for you. Then sleep well.

> *The blazing evidence of immortality*
> *is our dissatisfaction with*
> *any other solution.*
> Ralph Waldo Emerson
> *Journal*, July, 1855.

Chronophobia
(and other matters temporal)

> *The stars move still,*
> *time runs,*
> *the clock will strike,*
> *the Devil will come.*
> Christopher Marlowe
> *The Tragical History of Doctor Faustus*, 1604.

It's there: it ticks, it hums, it buzzes. You check it regularly, between tosses and turns, throughout the night. And while each time it tells a slightly different story, the basic plot is the same: at first it's still early, but that comfort zone gets chipped away, until that point when it's time to get serious about sleeping. Then all too soon it's only a couple of hours before you need to get up; the night has reached disaster level. You will definitely be tired and cranky all day. The clock has told you so.

Although there are books by sleep experts that recommend you never look at the clock during the night, I prefer to know how much time I have before the alarm goes off. Similarly, I like to know just how long I have been awake. If you decide to keep a sleep **journal**, it is important to gauge how many hours you have slept and how long you were awake during the night. You will also need to record the times you were awakened.

Don't, however, let the clock *control* your night. For one thing, clock-watching can be misleading: you may

20

not realize how much you have dozed between clock checks, thinking you have been awake the whole time. If you do awaken, once you note the time, or record it, forget about it. Go back to sleep. If it is close to the time the alarm is set to go off, congratulate yourself for sleeping so well.

But who can be drowsy at that hour
which freed us from everlasting sleep?
Or have slumbering thoughts at that time,
when sleep itself must end,
and, as some conjecture,
all shall awake again?
Sir Thomas Browne,
The Garden of Cyrus, 1658.

Don't think of the clock as your enemy. Once we had a very loud clock in our bedroom. I told my husband it was ticking off the seconds remaining in my life. How could anyone expect to sleep with such a reminder by their bed! We soon exchanged it, for a clock with lighted (quietly, I might add) numbers.

Look to the clock for information only, not as a basis for recriminations or judgements, good *or* ill. If you tire of checking it, and decide to get out of bed during the night, give yourself a time limit for staying up. Then stick to it. After that half hour, or hour, go back to bed, without checking the clock again.

Sometimes it helps to turn the clock face to the wall where you can't see it; if you have to reach, or even get out of bed to read it, you may just feel it isn't worth the effort. The better technique, though, is to train yourself to "forget" to check: if you awaken during the night, concentrate on falling back to sleep without worrying about what time it is, or how long you have been awake. Instead, enjoy the quiet of the night, enjoy the darkness, and sleep.

21

*At last the reins are twitched, the horses start,
and the sleigh bells, now violently shaken, strike
up their familiar music with a force that instantly
tears the gossamer of my dream. Again it is only
the shrill note of my alarm-clock.*

Sigmund Freud
The Interpretation of Dreams, 1900.

I used to wake myself up before the alarm clock
was scheduled to go off. Trained myself. I just couldn't
stand that invasive, repellant, buzzing. But turning off
the alarm brought with it the certain and unavoidable
fear of **oversleeping**. It was a less than ideal way to start
the day, waiting there in bed, nervous and anxious. And
coupled with a sleepless night, the combination could be
lethal to anyone's good nature. I came to find out later that
what I initially attributed to *chronophobia*, or fear of time,
was instead more a matter of taste: the way we are awakened in the morning *can* affect the way we approach the
new day. The reality is, too many of us wake up to the
sound of traffic, the train, or the crashing of trash cans as
the truck makes its early morning rounds. Perhaps the alarm
clock isn't so bad; you get to set the thing yourself, and
so have *some* control of the situation.

If you are anything like me, then, you can appreciate
that we live in a time unsurpassed for alarm clock alternatives. Want to wake up to the roar of ocean waves? How
about animal sounds of the rain forest? The call of songbirds? Maybe you would prefer a clock with a light that
slowly increases in wattage, imitating the dawn, allowing
your body to respond more naturally to its *circadian
rhythm*? For those that still see the alarm as an object of
disdain, the one encased in a shock absorbing enclosure,
allowing flights across the room, may be more your style.

Your sleep will not be filled with sweet dreams if, in
the early morning hours, you begin to dread that impending infernal noise. Turning off the alarm early may not be
the answer if you will just lie in bed, frustrated. On the

other hand, you could decide that waking up a little early, to **work out**, read the newspaper, or just have some time in the **quiet** of morning, may suit you. In any case, figuring out both your morning wake up or waking-during-the-night strategies can improve both the **quantity** and **quality** of your sleep.

Comfort

Other places do seem so cramped up and smothery, but a raft don't. You feel might free and easy and comfortable on a raft.
Mark Twain
The Adventures of Huckleberry Finn, 1884.

Is your sleep environment comfortable? In the physical sense, that is, not just as surroundings easily taken for granted. Be discerning: take a page from Goldilocks' book when considering your sleeping area.

Start with the bed. Sure, you're used to it, but could it be too hard or too soft for you? Are there spots beginning to sag? (The mattress, that is, not you.) Mattresses should be a compromise between tactile comfort and necessary support. As anyone who's slept on a too-soft hotel mattress can testify, the *"aaaahhhhh"* upon retiring can become an agonizing moan upon waking the next morning. For a modicum of comfort, a thicker pad or "featherbed", covering your sufficiently supporting mattress, may be what's needed

Is the ambient room temperature too hot, too cold, or just right? How about your personal temperature while under the covers? Sometimes changes in **weather** occur more readily than your adjustments in bed clothes; that down comforter that seemed so comfy just a week or two ago may now actually be *contributing* to your sleep problems.

Take a critical look at your **pillow**. Consider its height; neck and shoulder problems, as well as poor quality sleep, may result if it's too high or flat. A down pillow can be quite comfortable, as the feathers mold themselves to the shape and attitude of your head. But if it bothers you to wake up in the morning looking like Gumby, or you are allergic, you may want to look elsewhere. Many manufacturers claim sleep and overall health benefits for their pillows, based on their construction and filling material. Unfortunately, there is usually no opportunity to try before you buy. If you did invest in an expensive pillow and it isn't working out, give it to someone who might have better luck; don't let your precious sleep suffer for it.

Take your sheets seriously, especially if you sleep *au natural*. Fabrics with a higher thread count are generally the more comfortable to the touch. Natural fibers "breathe" better than man-made.

Think beyond the bed itself; extend your consideration of comfort to the entire room. Surround yourself with your favorite books, or **keepsakes**. Anything that makes you feel relaxed, secure, or safe is acceptable, so indulge yourself. Your bedroom is a "private" part of the house, so treat it accordingly: your only compromise need be with the person who shares your bed.

In future pages, we will be considering these aspects of your comfort in greater depth. For now, just keep in mind that when it comes to your bedroom, neither style nor grandeur nor luxury nor wealth is as important as comfort; and comfort is a critical component of sleep.

> *I went to the tree, and getting up into it, endeavoured to place myself so as that if I should sleep I might not fall...and having been excessively fatigued I fell fast asleep, and slept as comfortably as, I believe, few could have done in my condition, and found myself the most refreshed with it that I think I ever was on such an occasion.*
>
> Daniel Defoe
> *The Life and Adventures
> of Robinson Crusoe*, 1719.

Control

We do not what we ought;
What we ought not, we do;
and lean upon the thought
that chance will bring us through.
Nature with equal mind,
Sees all her sons at play;
Sees man control the wind,
the wind sweep man away.
Matthew Arnold
Empedocles on Etna, 1852.

You are under pressure, of course. It's a tough world, but you're tougher; you can pretty much handle anything that's thrown your way. If things don't work out, sometimes you get a little angry, (who wouldn't?), but if you spend enough time, and effort, somehow it will come out all right. It's almost always been that way.

How frustrating, then, that you can't sleep!

Sleep is not a contest. You don't need to win, to prevail; you just need to sleep. This is not a test of wills; after all, yours is the only will involved. Granted, the world *is* an increasingly challenging and confrontational place, but that is the world you will leave behind when you sleep. In order to do that, though, you must do the opposite of control: *you must let go.*

Think of the common expressions: to *drop off* to sleep, to *fall* asleep. I can remember, as a child, at times fairly *tumbling* into sleep, a free-falling, end-over-endless dive into a dark void. Perhaps giving up control is not, as an adult, so easily managed. But to achieve a restful sleep, a surrender to sleep must be negotiated.

Your feelings of frustration may stem from a lack of knowledge. This is not surprising, since for most readers, this book marks their first attempt at learning about sleep. If you find your need to control persists, direct it toward your *sleeplessness*: take what you learn here, and else-

25

where, and design a program for yourself. Think of yourself as an elite athlete: work at training and preparation, then trust in yourself, and your developed abilities, to manage your goal almost automatically.

Odds are, your first attempts won't be the end to your sleepless nights. Keep trying. But don't try *too* hard. Learn to let go, give in, and sleep. In peace.

Cry

Sleep, sleep, beauty bright,
dreaming o'er the joys of night.
Sleep, sleep: in thy sleep
little sorrows sit and weep.
William Blake
A Cradle Song, 1792.

While some may consider it the ultimate loss of control, I say: go ahead, have a good cry. Cry out of frustration, out of loneliness, out of worry. It need not be some actual **tragedy** that brings it about; and besides, (especially after a series of sleepless nights), tragedy can occur on a decidedly personal level. And although societal standards regarding such behavior may have you crying alone, in the privacy of your room, you shouldn't let them keep you from it altogether.

The benefits that can be found in tears lie as much in the result as the process. For those that can't remember those aftereffects personally, all you need to do is watch a small child to be reminded of the physical and emotional changes that can result from a good cry: it can be a remarkably cathartic, and physically taxing, exercise.

To put it in terms of the *Emotional Safety Handbook*: Don't equate a good cry with a system meltdown. It can, and should, instead be an emotional safety valve, relieving pressure before an impending explosion (or worse, an *implosion*).

Like any such device, however, it should be set to

go off well before the point of serious damage is reached. And, to be certain it's operating properly, it should be tested periodically.

Cure

There is no cure for life or death
save to enjoy the interval.
George Santayana
Soliloquies in England, War Shrines, 1922.

Your physician has confirmed it. You are not ill. And a clean bill of health from a medical professional should be a reason for celebration, even regarding your sleeplessness. It means that you can begin to find the *external* **cause(s)** of your problem sleep, and take the steps necessary to achieve relief.

Do not look to magic potions; sleep medications only help you to reach an otherwise natural state. Do not think of yourself as sick, in need of a cure. You are healthy, but temporarily compromised due to your lack of sleep. While you are not ill, you may be ill-equipped to handle the day after a sleepless night.

If you have been managing without the benefits of restorative sleep, think how much more talented and capable you will become with a full night of rest. Abandon your search for that ultimate "cure"; after all, you are not a piece of ham.

You are doing well. You are coping during a rough stretch. You are actively trying to learn to sleep peacefully, soundly, and regularly. You will manage it; you will sleep better. And you will be healthier for it.

What physic... can relieve, bear out, assuage,
or expel a troubled conscience?
A quiet mind cureth all.
Robert Burton
The Anatomy of Melancholy, 1621-1651.

Decision

You awaken in the middle of the night, feeling wide awake. What do you do?

Hard and fast rules regarding your actions often prove frustrating: there are times when your eyes first open that you know you will not be able to readily fall back to sleep; a dream may have disturbed you, or the caffeine from that late-night latte is starting to kick in.

With this in mind, there are times when it's best to immediately decide whether you will lie in bed, and try to fall back to sleep; or get up, and start another activity. The sooner you decide, and the less time you spend tossing and turning, the sooner you can derive benefits from either choice.

It's valid to use time to frame your decision. Give yourself twenty minutes, say, or half an hour, in order to fall asleep (but try not to watch the clock); then get up. What may seem like procrastination is, in fact, the opposite: you have committed to a sleep strategy that's manageable, and can avoid the anguish and ruminations over your next course of action that otherwise may trouble you for an indefinite (extended) period.

Once a decision was made,
I did not worry about it afterward.
Harry S. Truman
Memoirs, 1955.

If it's clear that sleep is unlikely, it is better to get out of bed rather than waiting. Eschew even the half-hour plan. Get up, have some warm milk or a cup of herbal tea, open a book. You may find yourself returning to sleep sooner than you anticipated: the book may be less entertaining than you remember, or you just may realize that lying in bed, warm and relaxed, is preferable to sitting up, in your robe, in the middle of the night.

You may decide to get up just long enough to make your rounds, to check the doors and windows, the weather outside, or check on the kids. Maybe you awaken just long enough to shake the lingering cobwebs from your bad dream.

In any case, once you decide your immediate course of action, you can rest easy, or, at least, *easier.* Appreciate the fact that you have decided, (no matter what the plan might be), and can avoid much of the recrimination and anxiety that uncertainty about your sleep can produce.

> *"Is this your decision, Monseigneur?" asked Aramis. "It is." "Irrevocably so?" Philippe did not even deign to reply. He gazed earnestly at the bishop, as if to ask him if it were possible for a man to waver after having once made up his mind.*
>
> Alexander Dumas
> *The Man in the Iron Mask,* 1850.

Decor

> *Infinite riches
> in a little room.*
> Christopher Marlowe, 1589.

Your surroundings *can* make a difference in your sleep, at least in terms of initiating it. Studies have shown that colors and decor can affect a person physically, as well as psychologically. If you have had trouble sleeping in the past, redecorating can not only result in an environment more conducive to rest, it can signal your taking a more active role in overcoming your sleep problems.

Certain colors —various pinks, aquas, and medium grays, for instance, have a reputation for their soothing qualities. The "Green Room", the backstage waiting area for stage performers, is so named for the color its walls were painted; the effect it produced on those awaiting their cues was one of relaxation and tranquility. The institutional green of government building interiors may have a similar calming, (if ultimately dehumanizing) effect; but I can't recommend holding that up as a model.

There are, however, no shortage of sources to help you get ideas for interior decorating. Just remember that magazine pictorials can be remarkably lacking when recreated in real life. And what works in a friend's place may not make the translation, either.

Instead, try this: the next time you're in a restaurant, museum, or other public place where you feel particularly comfortable or relaxed, take a moment to figure out what devices (including color combinations) are working to create this emotion. Though these are traditionally "neutral" spaces, they can, and should, have a distinct feel to them. Once you've identified them, decide what aspects (if any) could work for you in your bedroom.

But don't be bound strictly by tradition or convention, or what works for others; instead let your own personality dictate your efforts at redecorating. Experiment. Find the colors, patterns, prints, textures, and objects that appeal to you and indulge yourself spectacularly. Or, take a busy room down to its barest essentials. Spartan or ornate, it's up to you.

Paint each wall a different color, or a slightly different shade of the same color. Indulge in deep hued, saturated colors. Sponging or glazing walls can create multiple hues on the same wall, and the subtle gradations of each layer can produce a complex yet relaxing result. Perhaps you prefer light neutrals, and Navajo white is about as daring as you can manage. Then do it! In all your reckless glory, paint your walls Navajo white!

The goal is to create a *sleep environment* that both relaxes and rewards you. You should feel comfortable and calm in the entire room, not just in bed. And in learning about decor, don't miss the opportunity to learn about yourself, as well, as you work to extract the most joy, the most comfort, and the most sleep, possible from your environment.

Sleep came not near my couch– while the hours waned and waned away. I struggled to reason off the nervousness which had domin-ion over me. I endeavoured to believe that much, if not all of what I felt, was due to the bewildering influence of the gloomy furniture of the room– of the dark and tattered draper-ies, which, tortured into motion by the breath of a rising tempest, swayed fitfully to and fro upon the walls, and rustled uneasily about the decorations of the bed.

Edgar Allan Poe
Fall of the House of Usher, 1839.

Deep

The profound depth of the minister's repose was the more remarkable, inasmuch as he was one of those persons whose sleep, ordinarily, is as light, as fitful, and as easily scared away, as a small bird hopping on a twig.
Nathaniel Hawthorne
The Scarlet Letter, 1850.

You may have been a "deep sleeper" at some time in your past. Your life may be different enough now that you feel you can't allow it.

It might have been a single, isolated incident. A bur-glary or break in. A medical emergency. It may be the result of some negative conditioning that, though now a part of history, affects your sleep to this day. Battlefield experiences, or (risking redundancy) a bad marriage. It might not have even happened to you, but to a neighbor, or associate. It may even be a remnant of childhood, that time when experiences can be so deeply etched in your consciousness as to disturb you to this day. But whatever it is, it is compromising your sleep.

Determine if your concerns are justified. Are they realistic and rational, or are they representational of other matters in your life? Are they centered around your physical sleep environment, your surroundings, either immediate (your room or apartment) or extended (your town or city)?

Is the act of sleeping itself, the loss of consciousness and the vulnerability, the reason for your anxiety? Until the cause is identified *and you come to terms with it*, your sleep will suffer. Seek the help of a professional, if necessary. Even as progress is ongoing, work at breaking its connection to your sleep, which is necessary for both your mental and physical health.

Now I lay me down to sleep,
I pray the double lock will keep.
May no brick through the window break
and no one rob me 'till I awake.
Anonymous

Sometimes just the possibility of calamity is enough. What if you sleep through the smoke alarm, or your child's cries? You may overcompensate by sleeping less, or lighter. Unfortunately, what results is the opposite of what you intend: the debilitating effects of prolonged compromised sleep are profound. If you are responsible for someone's health and safety (even if it is just your own), you should recognize that sleep is not an indulgence, it is a necessity.

Assume you will wake up in an emergency. If you have to, condition yourself through your sleep **mantra** or pre-sleep **ritual** (dealt with in upcoming chapters) to awaken if the need ever arises.

And remember, even a sentry is relieved after a certain amount of time on watch.

Diet

Despite the recent evidence indicating a relationship between obesity and the incidence and severity of problem sleep, we're not necessarily saying a sleeker, thinner version of you will sleep better. But some basic concerns regarding the food you consume, particularly *what*, *when*, and *how much*, can play a significant role in the quality of your sleep.

What you eat can have a direct and almost immediate effect on your sleep, as anyone who has enjoyed a heavy dinner and a glass (or two) of wine can tell you. Meaty, rich, and fatty foods, in particular, can exacerbate the feelings of lethargy or fatigue that often accompany a large meal. Ironically, this effect may be short lived; since such foods take considerably longer to digest, disturbances to your digestion can mean disturbances to your sleep.

Similarly, spicy and unfamiliar foods can lead to a delayed onset heartburn that can interfere with, and even prevent your slumber. (We should note here that heartburn can be indicative of larger health problems, including a hiatal hernia or other gastric disorders, and should not be taken lightly; see your doctor for anything other than heartburn resulting from occasional overindulgence.)

On the other hand, certain foods may actually benefit your sleep. Higher levels of the amino acid *tryptophan* (found especially in dairy and poultry, accounting for that strong post-Thanksgiving dinner need-to-nap), vitamin B_6, folic acid and magnesium (all needed to metabolize *tryptophan*), and thiamine and zinc have been linked with elevated levels of *serotonin*. Increased levels of this chemical, produced by the body, have been associated with sleep. While evidence of a more direct connection between specific foods and improved sleep is still forthcoming, there just may be a scientific basis to that custom of a glass of warm milk before bed to bring about sleep.

33

*He gobbled them up... flesh, bones, marrow,
and entrails, without leaving anything
uneaten. ...but when the Cyclops had filled his
huge paunch, and had washed down his meal
of human flesh with a drink of neat milk, he
stretched himself full length upon the ground
among his sheep, and went to sleep.*
Homer
The Odyssey, 800 B.C.

*W*hen, and *how much*, you eat will also affect the
quality of your sleep on a given night.

*Is there no crumb of bread that you did keep?
I am so hungry that I cannot sleep.*
Chaucer
Canterbury Tales, 1380.

You don't need ongoing scientific research to tell you
that going to bed hungry can interfere with your sleep. A
light snack of easily digested food —fruits or other high
carbohydrate foods, can be preferable to "waiting 'till
breakfast" for the truly hungry. The no-calorie alternatives, a glass of water or cup of tea, can assuage your
hunger at least temporarily, but can count late night vis-
its to the bathroom among their disadvantages.

One connection between diet and sleep is fundamental: certain stages of the digestive process are not
designed to take place during sleep (or even in the horizontal position, for that matter). Give your digestive system too much to work on, or foods difficult to digest,
especially just before bed, and you risk disturbing your
rest.

Discomfort is discomfort, period. In sleep, like life
in general, moderation is the key. If you absolutely *must*
overindulge, at least plan your dinner time accordingly.
For those whose dining habits have spelled a dependence
on antacids, particularly those of the over-the-counter
variety, be advised that research is now drawing possible

34

links to a number of health problems related to their long term use; see your doctor about the suitability of other solutions to your condition.

> *For persons who dine contrary to custom experience much swelling of the stomach, drowsiness, and fullness; and if they take supper over and above, their belly is disordered; such persons will be benefited by sleeping after taking the bath, and by walking slowly for a considerable time after ...*
>
> Hippocrates
> *On Regimen In Acute Diseases*, 400 B.C.

We all know (or *should*, anyway) how much better our bodies work when they are kept in good condition; given the myriad physical problems stemming from being overweight, it should come as no surprise to count sleep problems among them. So, if you're still looking for a reason to get in shape (or yet *another* reason), add improved sleep to the list. You won't regret it, particularly when the benefits can be realized in both your waking and sleeping (and yes, even your *dining*) hours.

> *Do the feasters gluttonous feast?*
> *Do the corpulent sleepers sleep? have they lock'd and bolted doors?*
> *Still be ours the diet hard, and the blanket on the ground,*
>   *Pioneers! O pioneers!*
>
> Walt Whitman
> *Leaves of Grass*, 1855.

■ ■

Don't

We are not hypocrites in our sleep.
William Hazlitt
Table Talk, On Dreams, 1822.

Hold your tongue. Don't say it. Don't do it. Don't say what you feel simply *must* be said. Don't start that argument. Don't get that last word in. Not tonight. Not now, anyhow. Even though it may be *soooo* tempting.

Suddenly the house is quiet. The kids are finally asleep. The last guest has just left. The storm that has been brewing all night is about to be unleashed in a torrent of recriminations. Petty jealousies. Even insults.

Don't do it. In the name of all that is right and good, I beg you, DON'T DO IT. You will regret it the rest of the night as your "talk" drags on, mutating into something altogether different. You will regret it in the morning when you remember what you said when you were oh so tired and trying to end the whole "discussion".

Don't bring up the in-laws, the religion question, the money problems, at bedtime. Hold your tongue to avoid an extended late-night discourse that ends(?) with an apology just so you can get some rest before morning. Hold off. Count to ten. Count to a thousand. **Write** it down, if you have to. Just don't say it out loud, right now. You'll sleep better tonight and feel better tomorrow, if you don't.

In the morning, you'll say or do what must be done. In the light of day, it may not even be the concern it seemed to be just hours earlier. But even if it is, you'll be rested, and can better present your case with passion, and clarity. Good luck.

If you want to do something tonight
you'll be sorry for tomorrow,
sleep late.
Henny Youngman

Dreams

We are such stuff as dreams are made on,
and our little life is round with sleep.
William Shakespeare
The Tempest, 1611.

In your dreams you can travel to foreign lands, to territories not yet explored. You can meet and fall in love, with someone that needn't even exist. In your dreams you can be a different person, living a completely different life. You can see things and be things and do things that in the waking world would be impossible.

Father, O father! what do we here
In this land of unbelief and fear?
The Land of Dreams is better far
Above the light of the Morning Star.
William Blake

Though we are more concerned with sleep, and there is no shortage of books about dreams, their relationship is so linked as to bear inclusion here. Basically, you should look forward to sleep for the chance to dream. While scientists are uncertain over *why* we dream, their purpose, even whether they are innate or a result of our adaptation as a species, our brain assumes completely unique characteristics while we sleep. And even if you are one of those that cannot remember your dreams upon waking, you feel refreshed in the morning, in good measure, from the dreams of a good night's sleep.

Two Gates the silent house of Sleep adorn;
of polished ivory this, that of transparent horn;
True visions through transparent horn arise;
Through polished ivory pass deluding lies.
Virgil, *trans.* Dryden.
Aeneid, 19 B.C.

You may have realistic dreams, ones that include the minutiae of experiences from your day: a person, a pattern, a glimpse of color you hadn't even realized you noticed. Or they may operate on a larger scale, representing concerns from your waking life. In such cases, it can be a positive experience to dream about something that is troubling you; it can be a way to face it, adjust your attitude toward it, and even help you resolve it.

I had a recurrent dream in which I was being chased. It was set in the same forbidding, rocky canyon; often the same people played different roles. At first, I woke myself up when I found myself in these eerily familiar and troubling surroundings. Eventually, I learned to confront, then befriend, my would-be captors. The process took some time, and reflected a period in my life when I was juggling several projects and under tremendous pressure. This dream seemed to be a translation of that feeling, and gave me a chance to face, and deal with, my frustrations. Which doesn't mean this recurrent dream didn't scare me for a long time; some can be enough to make you dread turning out the light!

> *In the world of dreams I have chosen my part,*
> *To sleep for a season and hear no word*
> *Of true love's truth or a light love's art,*
> *Only the song of a secret bird.*
> A. C. Swinburne.

Other dreams, though, can exist purely for their fantastical aspect. You can find yourself in your own feature film, with control (or lack thereof) of casting, plot, and direction. You have access to vivid colors and surround sound *nonpareil*. Let go, imagine the most wonderful dream, and allow yourself to fully experience it. It is one of the few pleasures in life that you can indulge in completely and realize only benefits! If you are the type that finds yourself daydreaming during the day but has trouble sleeping at night, use the appeal of dreams as

38

part of a "carrot and stick" conditioning: you should look forward to bedtime and its freedom to dream for hours (uninterrupted) on end.

So sleep, and dream. Dream actively, dream enthusiastically, and rest your weary brain.

> *I've dreamt in my life dreams that have stayed with me ever after, and changed my ideas: they've gone through and through me, like wine through water, and altered the colour of my mind.*
> Emily Bronte
> *Wuthering Heights*, 1847.

Drop

It has been a remedy for sleeplessness since time immemorial. Take a warm bath before bed. And, truth is, it can be a surprisingly effective soporific.

But the reason *why* it works has taken a new twist. According to a recent study at the Cornell Medical Center in New York, it may be the sudden drop in body temperature *after* stepping out of the bath that's the cause of your sleepiness, more than the relaxing effects of the warm water. It mirrors a similar (if less dramatic) change your body undergoes during its transition to sleep.

So if your emergence into the cool air causes a **yawn** or two, take the hint; go to bed, and go to sleep.

> *There must be quite a few things a hot bath won't cure but I don't know any of them.*
> Sylvia Plath

Ebony

Amid the Cave, of Ebonye
a bedsted standeth bye,
And on the same a bed of downe
with keevering black doth lye,
In which the drowzye god of sleepe
his lither limbs doth rest.
Ovid; *trans.* Arthur Golding
Metamorphoses, 8 A.D.

Darkness. Emptiness. Ebony. The color black is unceasing, unknowable, and endless. Close your eyes. Pay no attention to the neon shapes and dots that may float by, under your closed eyelids; the field they dance on is our concern. Just shut your eyes, and shut down.

Black is the color of sleep, necessary for some to even attempt slumber. Physically, you can turn out the lights, pull the shades down, even hide under the covers, to achieve this desired state. Don a sleep **mask**, the night blindfold that came to mean "high society" in the movies, if you must. Or just close your eyes, to wrap yourself in a comforting envelope of night.

Hear, blessed Venus, deck'd with starry light,
In Sleep's deep silence dwelling, Ebon night,
Dreams and soft ease attend thy dusky train,
Pleas'd with the lenth'ned gloom and feastful strain...
Orphic Hymn

Embrace the darkness mentally, as well. Imagine the darkest night, shiny black olives, midnight gray thunderheads. Think of a warm, quiet, and enjoyable solitude. Drift off to sea on a lonely ship, without even the moon and stars to guide you. Swim in the deep water of a black bottomed pool. Imagine yourself in a theatre, waiting for the show to start. The lights have gone down, the curtain is up, and you have only to drop off, for the entertainment, your dreams, to begin.

40

Entertainment

The crowd are gone, the revellers at rest,
the courteous host, and all-approving guest,
Again to that accustomed couch must creep
Where joy subsides, and sorrow sighs to sleep...
Byron
Lara, 1814.

You've spent the evening out with friends, laughing and having a good time; you may still be stimulated by all the good conversation. Or you may be upset about the aftereffects of a bad date. You may have seen a thrilling movie, or a controversial play. In any case, the evening's activities have stayed with you to the degree that, even after returning home, you feel, "I couldn't possibly fall asleep now!"

After a while he glanced at the little clock that
was ticking on the mantelpiece. It was half-past
twelve. "It is funny," he said, "but it takes hours
to settle down to sleep after the theatre."
D.H. Lawrence
Sons and Lovers, 1913.

Sometimes it *does* help to go straight to bed. The **ritual** of readying for bed: changing your clothes, washing your face and brushing your teeth, can often be enough to prepare you, mentally and physically, for sleep.

At other times you might need to settle down a little. Watching TV is, for many, the ultimate soporific, but getting involved in a program or movie may put you in the situation of delaying sleep. Reading, especially a serious page-turner, may have the same result.

Winding down is particularly appropriate when the evening's activities have created a *physical* deterrent to your sleeping. An evening of dancing at a nightclub can bring your heart rate and blood pressure up to the levels of an aerobics class at the gym. Alcohol can work as a stimulant in lesser amounts, at higher levels, as a depressant; either situation is temporary, and the eventual change commonly interferes with sleep. Drinking and dancing can even bring about some *dehydration*, so make sure you drink enough (non-alcoholic) fluids. Especially loud concerts or nightclubs can leave your ears (as well as your entire body) feeling battered; *tinnitus*, or ringing of the ears, can last long after your revelry is done. I have found that classical **music**, or conversation, on the radio at low levels can work even better than silence to help "retune" my ears, and recalibrate not just my hearing, but my entire body.

If your troubled sleep traditionally demands extra attention, consider this when engaging in the evening's activities: make your last round a club soda, your after-hours espresso a decaf. Expect that what occurs late in your evening will have some effect on your slumber. Once home, the time it takes for a cup of tea (caffeine free, of course), or a warm bath (even if it's late), can repay your efforts with restful sleep.

> *After such an entertainment, he was wont to bathe, and then perhaps he would sleep till noon, and sometimes all day long.*
> Plutarch
> *Alexander*, 75 A.D.

Of course, there are those that work hard at play, and feel a night on the town is a treat for the senses not to be compromised. If you fall into this category you're likely to neither ask any quarter nor grant any. And if the evening involves *affaires l'amour*, well, all bets are off regarding sleep.

Escape

O magic sleep! O comfortable bird,
That broodest o'er the troubled sea of the mind
Till it is hushed and smooth!
Keats

You're trapped in a marriage or job you feel you can't get out of. You're in a place, a house, a city, you want to get away from. You're in debt, alone, overworked, underappreciated.

Most of all, you're tired. With all that's happening to you, it is hard to even find the time, let alone the inclination, to relax. So sleep becomes an afterthought, or worse: something not worth the effort. It is more comforting to stay awake watching bad television, or numb yourself with drugs or alcohol, than to go to bed and be alone, vulnerable, with your thoughts.

You're only contributing to your problems, though, with your lack of sleep. You are caught in a vicious cycle. The more tired you are, the less able you are to deal with your anxiety. However, the more anxious you are, the less you want to sleep. Obviously, this cycle must somehow be broken, but how?

Allow yourself an escape: when you turn off the lights, you turn off your anguish. Silence the mental voice that can be so demanding. Stop thinking of all that you are lacking, or protecting all that you have. Don't think about all you have to do, what is expected of you, or what is required. Save it for another time, when you are alert, rested, and up to the challenge.

> *At last his head fell heavily upon the cushion.*
> *Exhausted Nature had taken refuge in its last*
> *storehouse of vitality. It was half a sleep and*
> *half a faint, but at least it was ease from pain.*
> Arthur Conan Doyle
> *The Adventure of the Lion's Mane, 1926.*

Allow yourself the possibility that taking some time out is not ducking the matter. Grant yourself that inspiration may come to you after waking from a good night's rest, that a solution may be even more evident in the light of day. Stop contemplating, worrying, thinking; at least while you're in bed at night.

Even a fast moving stream has *eddies*, calm pools of still water. The easiest way to find the eddies in your busy life may be to create them yourself; bed time is an ideal time for their establishment.

The ability to reduce anxiety is beneficial, both for your mental and physical health. By practicing it in pursuit of sleep, it may translate to your waking hours, as well.

Eventually

It may not seem like it at the time, as you toss and turn for what seems an eternity, but eventually *you will fall asleep*. It may be just before the alarm goes off (darn!); or it may be as you lie on the couch after work, with your feet up, after a long day at the office (not recommended).

Eventually, you will sleep. It's hard to imagine sometimes, I know, but it happens, with remarkably few exceptions, to *everyone, every night*. You're one of those noteworthy exceptions, you say? While I may grant you the exceptional nature we all possess as individuals, the sheer numbers, and the way we're biologically wired, make a strong case to the contrary.

Eventually; maybe not this moment, and maybe not when you would prefer it, but eventually, you will fall asleep. Take comfort (and a lesson) in the fact that anxiety over whether or not sleep will happen can only delay, not prevent it.

Eye of the Storm

An age employed in edging steel
can no poetic raptures feel...
No shaded stream, no quiet grove
can this fantastic century move.
Philip Freneau
Poems, 1795.

All hell is breaking loose. Your job, your kids, your spouse, your in-laws, are all conspiring to make your daily existence as difficult as possible. Your secretary quit, your roommate doesn't have the rent, your dog is sick. Lately your ulcer is acting up, and now you feel a headache coming on. What can a person do?

Sometimes it's best to do nothing.

"Nothing?" you say, "but how will I ever make it through the holidays if I'm not the family mediator? How will I get promoted if I can't push this deal past Johnson in accounting? How will I pay next month's rent?"

It is easy, sometimes, to get so caught up in **responsibilities** that you lose sight of the efficiency of your actions. In concentrating so on the furious paddle upstream, you miss the fact that some things can best be obtained simply by waiting on shore for them to eventually float past.

But with all that is going on around you, demanding your attention, turning you this way and that, it may be more appropriate to use a quite different illustration.

The power of a hurricane is undeniable. It generates winds of tremendous speed, and is a furious force of destructive energy. Yet at its center it is still, and quiet.

Imagine yourself in, imagine yourself *as*, the eye of the storm. You are inside it; it is not inside you. Breathe deeply, and think of all the personal dramas being played out similarly; as *around* you, not *inside* you. They are close, yes, but at the same time removed from your direct experience.

45

The eye of the storm offers a unique perspective. You have not *removed* yourself from all that is destructive and distractive around you; quite the contrary: you are as closely involved as ever before. But instead of being swept up in the rush of energy that can hinder, even prevent, efficiency, you see things more clearly. You can develop a workable plan for action. You can separate important concerns from the incidental debris that gets sucked up as the storm moves along.

Let the others be tumultuous and bitter, let them fight and bicker over incidentals. You will choose actions that are productive and efficient. By putting yourself directly in the middle of the chaos, you find order.

> *I perhaps ought to have met the storm,*
> *had I thought myself capable*
> *of resisting it.*
> Rousseau
> *Confessions,* 1766-1770.

You are the eye of the storm. The center. And when you lie in your bed at night, the hush that envelopes you is restful and restorative. The concerns of the world are still there, spinning wildly; and while you are aware of them, you don't have to deal with them. Not now. For a while, if you choose, you can laugh at them, at the frantic actions of those involved, or marvel at their complexities, at the strange way the world operates.

Or you can just relax. And sleep.

> *As long as skies are blue,*
> *and fields are green,*
> *Evening must usher night,*
> *night urge the morrow...*
> Percy Bysshe Shelley
> *Adonais,* 1821.

■ ■

Eyes

Twas dead of night, when weary bodies close
Their eyes in balmy sleep and soft repose...
Virgil
Aeneid, 29-19 B.C.

As hard as it may be to function after a sleepless night, the worst part may be looking as bad as you feel. Bloodshot eyes. Droopy eyelids. Puffy bags underneath. You may find yourself looking in a mirror in the morning and seeing the image of your grandmother, (regardless of which gender you are!).

One concern surrounding the appearance of your eyes is of the "chicken and egg" variety: are your eyes showing the strain from lack of sleep, or are you having trouble sleeping because of eye strain?

If your eyes bother you during the day, then eye problems may also be interfering with your falling asleep. Get yourself a complete eye exam. Chances are it has been a while since your last one. Make certain, especially if your age warrants it, that the exam includes a test for glaucoma. If the doctor gives you a clean bill of health, there are still a number of things you can do to ease the strain on your eyes.

If your **work** involves the use of a computer monitor or similar visual display, an anti-glare attachment can reduce glare *on* the screen and certain ultraviolet frequencies *from it*. Sit back at least 24 inches from the screen, and resist the tendency to lean or slump forward. Take breaks; if not of the full, around-the-watercooler variety, at least periodically turn your attention to a task that doesn't involve the monitor. And even while you are using it, remember to shift your vision away from the screen, to focal points both nearer and farther away, regularly throughout the session.

Practice this "eye-sometric" exercise: hold your extended forefinger about one foot from your eyes. Bring it into focus. Now shift your focus to the background. Finger. Background. Move your finger to arms length and bring it slowly toward you, stopping every few inches for the finger/background shift. This ability to shift focus commonly deteriorates with age.

So does the amount of moisture your eyes produce; keep some "bottled tears" or similar natural, low chemical eye drops on your desk (and use them regularly) to help prevent eye strain.

You may be one of those whose eyes show the affects of strain in their appearance. If so, some tried-and-true remedies include placing cold sliced cucumbers (please resist the urge to use hamburger dill pickles) or moistened tea bags upon your closed eyes. Or drape a cold, wet washcloth across them to soothe, darken the room, and reduce the associated puffiness, as well. Those plastic masks filled with a thermal fluid are readily available and reasonably priced; remember that most should not be frozen, only refrigerated. Be careful, too, when you take it off, not to leave it on the floor near the bed; one misstep in the morning can mean the end of both the mask and your white carpet!

Remember, we close our eyes to cue our body to sleep. If you feel you have to close them because *they* need rest or relief, you may find yourself unable to sleep, or initiating a confused sleep cycle.

Take care of your eyes; they work hard for you. Close them and sleep your well-deserved sleep.

Come, heavy sleep...
And close up these my weary weeping eyes,
Whose spring of tears doth stop my vital breath,
And tears my heart with sorrow's sigh-swollen cries...
John Dowland

Family Bed

If you are unfamiliar with this term, it means YOUR CHILDREN SLEEP WITH YOU, IN YOUR BED. Boy, can this ever affect your sleep.

> *Familiarity breeds contempt—*
> *and children.*
> Mark Twain
> *Notebooks*, 1835–1910.

It can affect the time you go to bed. Your children will want you to go to bed with them, and you may find yourself lying in bed (albeit temporarily) at an hour when sleep is, for you, impossible. If they are night owls, or have had the advantage of an afternoon nap, they may have you pleading with them to turn out the light because you just can't read another bedtime story. Then you have to put up with their **fidgeting** and restlessness because *they aren't tired!* I know, the parent is the boss. Try explaining that to a tired two year old.

> *Backward, turn backward,*
> *O Time, in your flight.*
> *Make me a child again*
> *just for tonight!*
> Elizabeth Akers Allen
> *Rock Me To Sleep*, 1860.

The family bed will also affect the **quality** of your sleep. Children are "active" sleepers more often than adults; you may be kicked and shoved throughout the night, until you find yourself perched at the very edge of the bed. At the same time, you may be worried all night that *they'll* fall out.

You may have a child that awakens often. They are hungry, thirsty, or scared. You will have to wake up too.

49

And too often you may find yourself remaining wide awake after they have comfortably, snugly, and quite successfully, gone back to sleep. Of course, no parent is completely immune to this, whether the child is in their bed or not.

There was a time when our son suffered dangerously high fevers, with resultant febrile seizures. Due to their sudden, unpredictable nature, we decided that, for his goodwill and our own peace of mind, we would have him sleep in bed with us. We learned a great deal in sleeping with (both literally and figuratively) our little ball o'fire.

First, determine the optimal time for your child(ren) to go to bed. Try to teach them to fall asleep without your presence; this will simplify your life and help greatly when they make the transition to their own bed. Since they cannot be up later than you, if you find you're staying up to accommodate them, stop. Make certain of their comfort and needs before the lights go out (and make sure they're aware that you've asked); while it can't prevent, it can reduce the need for drinks of water or extra blankets in the course of the night.

Between the dark and the daylight,
When the night is beginning to lower,
Comes a pause in the day's occupations,
That is known as the Children's Hour.
Henry Wadsworth Longfellow
The Children's Hour, 1860.

Many families maintain some aspect of the family bed, whether by design or not. Many that would never accept the idea in concept have a remarkably liberal "early morning visitor" program in effect. Others believe strongly in the family bed as a way to foster love and closeness as a family. The idea of parents sleeping with their small child, or children, has been around for thousands of years, in cultures throughout the world. If it is important to you, do not give up the idea of the family bed due to outside

50

pressure. Because there *will* be pressure: it seems anyone that's had children (or *been* one, for that matter) has an opinion of how children should be raised. When it turned out that my son's presence in our bed (we believe) may have saved his life, it became impossible to convince us that it would be bad for him, no matter how many kiddie bedroom gifts he received from well-meaning grandparents and friends, or how many frowns of disapproval from others.

The family bed can be somewhat (gross understatement) inconvenient. Other times, it can feel like a nightly slumber party. With an infant, early morning feedings can be decidedly easier, though the parental involvement *will* be more shared. Once our son outgrew the situation, he was in his own room. But for almost four years our son was on my side of the bed, for me to watch over and nurture. How wonderful it is to wake up in the smooth, chubby arms of your loving child! The smell of their curly hair, warm cheeks, and baby breath are unforgettable. And every morning he had to hug me upon waking, whether he liked it or not. He never came between my husband and me, physically or emotionally, and all of us woke up happy in the knowledge that he had passed another safe night.

Whether you choose to have your small child(ren) sleep with you or not, be strong; follow your own instincts as a parent. You'll sleep better for it.

> *"I know where it blooms," said a happy mother, who came with her lovely child to the bedside of the queen. "I know where the loveliest rose in the world is. It is seen on the blooming cheeks of my sweet child, when it expresses the pure and holy love of infancy; when refreshed by sleep it opens its eyes, and smiles upon me with childlike affection."*
>
> Hans Christian Andersen
> *The Loveliest Rose In the World*

Fidgeting

"Damnation! Why do you keep fidgeting—
why don't you go to sleep?" his brother's voice
called to him.

Leo Tolstoy
Anna Karenina, 1876.

Tossing. Turning. First on one side, then the other. Maybe you've even been told (or told yourself) to stop, already! But how to stop, especially when you aren't sure how it began or what keeps it going. Face it, the last time any of us was truly comfortable was in the womb, and there's none of us going back! Restless may equal REST + LESS; but what you need is to rest *more*. Consider that your fidgeting may be not a *symptom* of your sleeplessness, but a *cause*.

Relax. Don't turn or squirm immediately over a temporary discomfort, some irritating signal that your body has sent from an extremity. Instead, turn it to your advantage: use that itch, that twinge, as a way to focus. By not *automatically* reaching for relief, you can consider the nature and extent of each physical need, then use your mind to calm each area variously demanding your attention. Itchy calf? Don't reach, at least not immediately. Lay still, and try to send a dose of anesthetizing relaxation to it, a spreading wave that emanates from that spot. Do the same for anything else that has you squirming.

A physical need does not always require a physical response. It will take some practice, but with time, the only person more thankful than your bed partner may be you.

I found myself weary and yet wakeful, tossing
restlessly from side to side, seeking for the
sleep which would not come.

Arthur Conan Doyle
The Hound of the Baskervilles, 1901.

Firmness

If you were talked into a new vacuum cleaner by a door to door salesman, or another set of tickets to the Policeman's Ball by a telemarketer, you may find yourself lying awake in bed, kicking yourself, instead of sleeping. How about having just been lured into another deadly boring social commitment by a well-meaning friend or relative? "I should have been more firm; should have just said '*No*'", you think to yourself, while lying in the dark in the middle of the night.

If your will is not strong during the daylight hours, you open yourself up to the regrets and doubts that always seem to come creeping in with the darkness. The strength of your resolve could come under scrutiny as you lie there, reliving the day. Doubting your abilities to handle a given situation may even find you questioning your capabilities as a sleeper!

Stand up for yourself. Be polite (always), but *be firm*: in your dealings with others, and in the decisions you make for yourself. Resolve to stand firm; have confidence in the choices you make and your abilities. You will sleep better for it.

> *For human nature*
> *is as surely made arrogant*
> *by consideration, as it is awed*
> *by firmness.*
> Thucydides
> *History of the Peloponnesian War*, 413 B.C.

And, on an altogether different consideration of firmness, how is that mattress of yours? Soft and lumpy? Hard, but springy? Quite often the reason for your sleeplessness can be found directly beneath you. Your bed. In particular, your mattress. If you are sleeping (or rather, not sleeping) on an old, worn mattress, it just might be time for a change. Mattresses have a definite lifespan, one relative to the quality of their construction. If that special occasion (like getting a place of your own, or getting married) that prompted you to purchase your current mattress is now ancient history, it may be time to consider a new one.

Read about them, compare methods of construction, but don't select a mattress without giving it the Goldilocks test: lie down on each, until you find the one that is "just right"; then stay there for a while. After all, you are the one that will be sleeping on it every night for years, not the commissioned salesperson. A mattress is a major purchase; you are allowed to make a pest of yourself in the showroom.

> *The newcomer went to the bunks and inspected the blankets; he lifted up the mattress, and then dropped it with an exclamation. "My God!" he said, "that's the worst yet."*
>
> Upton Sinclair
> *The Jungle*, 1906.

When shopping, don't rule out "alternative" sleep systems; a fluid, air, or other support medium may be just what you need. If you opt for a conventional mattress, don't forget to turn it regularly, as the manufacturers recommend. It's like changing the oil in your car: while it will still work without doing it, it becomes a question of how well and for how long.

Whether it's a simple futon with its hard wooden frame, or an elaborate waterbed with its gentle waves, find the bed that best suits your taste, your lifestyle, your **decor**, but most important, *your back*! No matter what your choice, a firm, comfortable mattress can help you sleep more deeply, and soundly.

Stand firm, in your pronouncements and decisions. Lie firm, on your mattress. And sleep well. You deserve it after all your hard work just getting through today...regardless of what your day was like.

Flowers

...Silent moves
The feet of angels bright;
Unseen they pour blessing,
And joy without ceasing,
On each bud and blossom;
And each sleeping bosom.
William Blake

Fresh flowers. No matter how jaded or hard boiled you think you are, the essence of flowers can, in turn, stimulate almost to intoxication, or enervate to debilitation. Fortunately, the effects of fresh cut flowers are far more subtle. Try roses in a vase by the bed, or bracts of lavender on your night stand; two types of flowers long associated with sleep.

The currently popular phenomenon of *aroma therapy* has been around in its most natural form for centuries. Various native cultures have held the night blooming *Datura* as sacred, believing that its blossoms, placed near the head on your pillow at night, would open the door to adventurous dreams. Not surprising, really, given the psychoactive (and dangerously toxic) alkaloid compounds they contain. Similar tribute has been given to flowers of the related *Belladonna*, and *Nightshade* families.

A *night blooming Jasmine* is more my style. That or the "curry plant" (*Helichrysum italicum*) that we've sown along our paths: when our legs brush by them, particularly on a warm summer evening, the aroma almost makes us swoon.

Which, as we've talked about, can cause problems for people with allergies. But there is more than just fragrance to cut flowers. It is the dried parts of the Chamomile *flower*, for instance, that produces the tea favored for its sleep producing powers. And many types of flowers, from exotic orchids and lilies to the lowly (regal?)

55

daisy, have an appeal that goes beyond fragrance; their beauty and natural aspect lend an air of tranquility to our lives, helping us on our way to a more peaceful sleep. You can't ask much more, can you? From a plant, I mean.

The image of love, that nightly flies
To visit the bashful maid, that sighs
Steals from the Jasmine flower, in the shade,
Its soul, like her,
The hope, in dreams, of a happier hour
That alights on misery's brow,
Springs out of the silvery almond flower,
That blooms on a leafless bough.
Then haste we, maid,
To twine our braid,
Tomorrow the Dream of flowers will fade.

T. Moore
Lalla Rookh:Nourmahal's Song

Gentle

Oh Sleep!
it is a gentle thing...
Samuel Taylor Coleridge
The Ancient Mariner, 1798.

Lead a gentle life, and enjoy a gentle sleep. A day spent cursing the dawn, cutting off others on the expressway, complaining about service, and generally being cruel, coarse, or crude does not bode well for a good night's sleep.

O sleep! O gentle sleep!
Nature's soft nurse,
how have I frighted thee,
that thou no more wilt weigh my eyelids down
and steep my senses in forgetfulness?
William Shakespeare
Henry the Fourth, 1598.

Government

Politics make strange bedfellows.
Charles Dudley Warner, 1870

You are so angry. They've done it again. How could the Mayor/Councilman/Senator/President do such a thing? What were they thinking? Now that you mention it, how did they even get elected? What's wrong with people?

It is a curious phenomenon, that tendency to see things with utmost clarity only after the room is darkened. (Of course, that few minutes of eleven o'clock news you watched before bed *might* have something to do with it). Unfortunately, in recognizing the problem so suddenly, the urgency to act can also be unsurpassed. Someone ought to write a letter, start a petition, make some phone calls. Maybe it should even be you.

Perhaps you *are* right. Those jerks just can't run things properly. Your passion is admirable, your frustration understandable. But hold on. While you are lying in bed, ruminating and fuming, mentally writing your letter, getting your petition signed, maybe even going over your acceptance speech, the powers that be are *sleeping*.

I tell you folks,
all politics is apple sauce.
Will Rogers
The Illiterate Digest, 1924.

Or not sleeping; which may explain why elected officials age so while in office. So why begin your efforts cranky and tired, when tanned, rested and ready (and yes, cranky) is what's called for. Get some rest. Wait until morning, then go ahead: start making your phone calls, (rational ones, please), and learn more about the issues that concern you. You *should* be involved, *should* be

57

aware of the decisions, on every level, that affect us all. By working to change things for the better, and realizing your contribution in doing so, it is less likely you will be lying in bed at night with your fists clenched in anger.

Keep in mind that the words you compose after a good night's sleep will be more effective than those rehearsed in bed in the dark. The plan for action will be more realistic, and the chances for success far greater.

But be aware, too, of the dangers inherent in such involvement. Bringing about change can mean taking on the system, with its own, unique, and quite formidable brand of frustration; don't let yourself become vulnerable to it. Be wary, but be glad that you possess enough passion to test the process.

> *He is the happy warrior*
> *of the political battlefield.*
> Franklin D. Roosevelt
> *Nominating speech for Al Smith,*
> *Democratic National Convention,* 1924.

Go ahead, feel strongly about the political system, about injustice and inequality, about the state of things today. Then come up with positive, effective, and nonviolent solutions. Who knows, your efforts may even help others to sleep better at night.

> *There's just one rule for politicians all over the world: Don't say in Power what you say in Opposition; if you do, you only have to carry out what the other fellows have found impossible.*
> John Galsworthy
> *Maid in Waiting,* 1931.

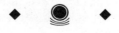

Green

*The mountain-tops are asleep, and the mountain-gorges, ravine and promontory:
Green leaves, every kind of creeping things
On the breast of the dark earth, sleep...*
Alcman, *trans.* W. Headlam

Surround yourself with living plants for their undeniable physical benefits. They help turn the used-up exhaust of our respiration into fresh, usable air. They filter out pollutants and counteract the effects of many airborne toxins. They can even make a room quieter. It follows that having healthy house plants in your home, and in your bedroom in particular, can help you to sleep.

But the advantages of greenery can reach beyond the physical actions of the plants themselves, and beyond the boundaries of your room. There can be tremendous emotional and psychological benefits to those that choose to cultivate a relationship with *florae*. It is, after all, part of our "natural" state. And while it is not for everyone, those that do take to tending a garden, no matter how large or small, commonly describe working among plants as "relaxing" or "meditative". Time, along with other concerns of daily life, seems somehow diminished while you are in communion with nature.

Find a public garden in your city, and sign up for some planting space (or at least join the waiting list, behind the others already aware of the benefits). Work in your yard, if you are lucky enough to have some land, no matter how small and shady a patch it may be.

For your convenience, choose plants suited to your region, and relative to your available time and inclination for work: if you want to sit and commune, rather than prune, keep that in mind. Similarly, if planting for cut flowers rather than table vegetables is more your style, so be it.

Plant an herb garden on your balcony, fire escape, or in a window box, if space is limited; you could even sow some of the many **herbs** favored for their sleep benefits.

Surround your home, and your life, with nature. It can be as simple as a walk in the park, or a weekend out of the city. The benefits of nature are available to anyone that takes the time and makes the effort to seek it out, no matter how "urban" their existence. Do so. You will sleep better for it. Guaranteed.

> *There is, perhaps, no solitary sensation so exquisite as that of slumbering on the grass or hay, shaded from the hot sun by a tree, with the consciousness of a fresh but light air running through the wide atmosphere, and the sky stretched overhead upon all sides. Earth, and heaven, and a placid humanity seem to have the creation to themselves. There is nothing between the slumberer and the naked and glad innocence of nature.*
>
> Leigh Hunt

> *There in close comfort by some brook,*
> *Where no profaner eye may look,*
> *Hide me from Day's garish eye,*
> *While the bee with honey'd thigh,*
> *That at her flowery work doth sing,*
> *And the waters murmuring,*
> *With such concert as they keep,*
> *Entice the dewy-feathered sleep.*
> *And let some strange mysterious dream*
> *Wave at his wings in airy stream*
> *Of lively portraiture display'd,*
> *Softly on my eyelids laid,*
> *And, as I wake, sweet music breathe*
> *Above, about, or underneath,*
> *Sent by some spirit to mortals good,*
> *Or the unseen genius of the wood.*
>
> John Milton
> *Il Penseroso*

Guilt

" 'I have to make a clean breast of it all. You can hang me, or you can leave me alone. I don't care a plug which you do. I tell you I've not shut an eye in sleep since I did it, and I don't believe I ever will again until I get past all waking...'"
A. Conan Doyle
The Adventure of the Cardboard Box, 1893.

How can you sleep, after what you have done? How will you sleep again, *ever*? How can you even live with yourself? All very good questions, just the type of questions to ask IF YOU NEVER WANT TO SLEEP AGAIN!!!

If you are suffering from guilt, you cannot expect to sleep; at least, not as well as you should. After all, such expressions describing the "sleep of the innocent" and the "sleep of the guilty" developed for a reason. Alone, in the dark, with minimal outside distractions, the mind is most vulnerable to those emotions it has tried to suppress throughout the day.

So save it. Take that guilt (and its close relative, regret), and put it somewhere far away, lest it loom over your bed like some giant, black cloud. No matter how wrong you have been, and you may have been *very* wrong, you still need to get a good night's rest. Save it all for **morning**, when your mind is clear. You won't learn anything from your midnight ruminations that you don't already know, and denying yourself much needed sleep may only serve to make you angry and resentful, perhaps even toward the person(s) you have wronged!

For that middle-of-the-night, "what have I done?" quick fix, take steps to minimize the flood of emotion: breathe deeply to relax and loosen those chest muscles so affected by stress. Engage in some **progressive relaxation**. Have a good **cry**, or a pillow punching session. Sit down and **write** an apology, whether you intend to mail it or not. As a last resort, rationalize your actions to the point where you can sleep. Don't let guilt drag you down. At least not tonight.

> *The harrowing remorse robbed her of her sleep. She never broke the fierce silence under which she laid herself, when she opened her mouth, it was only to cry out her crime before God and man.*
> Stendahl
> *The Red and the Black,* 1830.

In the morning, wake up with the resolve to make things right. Know that rationalizing your actions to assuage guilt is a lot like mowing a weed: though it looks better temporarily, it won't be long before it returns, bigger than ever. Plan the steps you will take to deal with the problem; it may begin with mailing the letter you wrote the night before, or finally making that call.

Above all, learn from your actions. Vow not to repeat your mistakes. The more guilt you harbor, the more vulnerable you make yourself to future moral compromises. Do whatever's in your power to make things right. Then learn to live with it, and live to learn from it. And sleep.

> *Let not the sluggish sleep*
> *Close up thy waking eye,*
> *Until with judgment deep*
> *Thy daily deeds thou try;*
> *He that one sin in conscience keeps*
> *When he to quiet goes,*
> *More vent'rous is than he that sleeps*
> *With twenty mortal foes.*
> William Byrd

Hammock

*How captivating is a Peruvian lady, swinging in
her gaily-woven hammock of grass, extended
between two orange-trees, and inhaling the
fragrance of a choice cigarro!*

Herman Melville
Typee, 1846.

You always seem to fall asleep in the one in Joe's
backyard, or out at the cabin on the lake. It might not be
just the warm sun or the gentle breezes lulling you to
sleep; that contraption you're sleeping on may be contributing more to your slumber that you realize. For while
you probably put sleeping in a hammock in the novelty
category, many cultures around the world use them as
their primary sleep system.

There is something about the type of support it offers: like giant arms cradling your body. A well made hammock with a proper fit makes you feel almost weightless,
with no individual support points on your body to de-
stroy the illusion. In summer, or in warmer climes, the
flow-through ventilation it offers is unsurpassed. And of
course, with your every movement, there's that gentle
rocking motion...

Try it in the one- or two- person variety, freestand-
ing or strung between two sturdy trees or posts. Enjoy
the relaxing qualities that sleeping outdoors in a hammock can bring, even if it's just on your balcony. Or, if
you're adventurous enough, go native! Bring that hammock inside (more than likely in a corner, and make certain it's anchored into the studs, and not just wall material), put on the *Polynesian Strings* for a bit of added at-
mosphere, and sleep!

*...each got into his hammock to taste the sweets
of a tranquil sleep.*

Johann Wyss
Swiss Family Robinson, 1813.

Headache

A simple headache could be all that lies between you and sleep. "Nothing simple about this!" you lament, as you battle your second migraine in as many weeks. And, to be certain, headaches, like any body pain, can be an indication that a more serious health problem exists. You should see your doctor to rule out any such conditions. However, given the number of analgesics available, it's safe to say few of us have been spared this all-too-human malady.

Which doesn't mean you have to suffer, especially if your headache is interfering with your sleep. The first step, if at all possible, is to try to determine its cause. This may be harder than it sounds, particularly if your headache is recurrent, but as a general health practice it is far more effective to treat causes, rather than symptoms.

Stress related headaches, in particular, can often be relieved with breathing, or other relaxation exercises. Those included in this book are but an introduction, so if you find yourself responding to such methods, we encourage you to go further.

Simple accupressure techniques may also help, such as pressing firmly but gently with your thumb and forefinger on the bridge of your nose, at the corners of your eyes, for at least 20 seconds. Pinching/kneading the tip of the right big toe, or pinching gently the middle of your upper lip, may also provide relief. (It can't hurt to *try*, anyway.)

Tension headaches, especially those emanating from the region where the head and neck join, may be the result of stress, or bad posture. A rolled up towel, placed under your neck while you lie on your back, can take some of the pressure off the muscles and help to restore the natural curve of your spine in that area. Don't make the roll too large, though, especially at the start. And if you happen to fall asleep, (great!) just remove the towel, roll over, and continue to snooze.

A "nonspecific" headache can often be helped by scalp massage. Use your fingertips in a shampooing motion, with enough firm pressure to make the scalp "slip" against the skull. The relaxation of the scalp muscles and increase in blood flow to the area can be enough to bring relief. This is even more effective (and enjoyable) if someone else administers it. Sometimes a hot shower, with cool or cold water to finish, sets up an "expansion/contraction" of the circulatory system that can also help you feel better. While this may not seem like the best middle-of-the-night solution, neither is lying there, in pain.

Sometimes headaches are a result of dehydration. Drink up: not just at bedtime, but during the course of the day. If a need for caffeine or nicotine is the cause of your nighttime headache, though, we can't recommend assuaging that craving.

If all else fails, you may have to resort to approved medications or herbal supplements. Take them strictly as recommended. Even over-the-counter headache remedies should be taken moderately, as directed; and as a problem sleeper, be advised: many "plain" aspirins contain enough caffeine to disturb your sleep, so read the label.

Any situation involving headaches should be temporary. Don't allow it to become anything but. **Pain** is part of the body's warning system. Answer its call first, take the steps necessary to relieve it, then sleep.

When you're lying awake
with a dismal headache,
and repose is tabooed by anxiety,
I conceive you may use
any language you choose
to indulge in, without impropriety.
Sir William S. Gilbert, (Gilbert & Sullivan)
Iolanthe, 1882.

Herbs

...there growes of Poppye store
With seeded heades, and other weedes
innumerable more,
Out of the milkie jewce of which
the night doth gather sleepes,
And over all the shadowed earth
with darkish dew them dreepes.
Ovid; *trans*. Arthur Golding

For thousands of years the physic powers of certain plants have been associated with sleep. From those inducing it to those preventing it (along with a varied assortment of those simulating, prolonging, and enhancing), humans have long looked to the world of *florae* for assistance with sleep. At no time, however, has the connection between herbs and sleep been explored as much as now. For despite the explosion of pharmaceutical developments in recent years, more people than ever are looking to the natural benefits of plants, in particular, herbs, as an aid to sleep.

The manner in which these herbs may be used are almost as varied as the plants themselves. In their most natural form, leafy or flowering herbs may be collected and placed around the house, with benefits realized merely by their proximity. Cut *lavender* and *rose* blossoms, for instance, have long been noted for their relaxing quality. In other cases, culinary or medicinal herbs are consumed: either raw or cooked, alone or as an added ingredient. That cup of *chamomile* tea sweetened with *honey* that Grandma might have recommended, for instance, represents two traditional, natural sleep inducers.

The oils of herbs and plants may also be extracted by a variety of techniques, producing a concentrated essence, or *essential oil*. These oils may be used in massage, baths, inhalations (either in steam or through a bowl-like burner or infuser) or as a perfume or fragrance. Essential oil mixtures to relieve insomnia or nervous tension might include those based on *vetiver,* sometimes called "nature's tranquilizer", or blending *neroli* with *ylang-ylang* oil and *sandalwood,* for instance; or feature *lemon-balm* with the aforementioned classics, *lavender* and *rose* oils.

Other plants and herbs with relaxing or sleep inducing attributes include: some commonly used by cooks everywhere, *sweet marjoram* and *basil*; the Chinese herbalists' *ginseng*; brewers' *hops*; the exotic *passionflower* fruit; the common *California poppy* and *primrose*; the much maligned *cannabis*; and your pet's personal favorite: *catnip.* Add to the list *kava-kava, valerian, skullcap, spikenard, calamint, benzoin* and *petitgrain,* and we still haven't included them all.

What to make of all of this? What you will. I place the use of herbal remedies in the same realm as pharmaceuticals: as a resort for those that have exhausted other, more internal, and more manageable, means of sleep.

Like all medications, contraindications abound; some cannot be taken with other herbs, while others are most effective only when taken in conjunction with a complementary herb. Some, like *camphor* and *eucalyptus*, are soothing and relaxing at certain doses, but stimulating at a just slightly higher level. Nuances can extend to other areas *(neroli* can be much more soothing than *bergamot,* for instance, though they are similar formulas), further confusing the issue. Adding to the difficulties, non-controlled production of essential oils can lead to varying dose and quality standards; quite often essential oils are adulterated with other (cheaper) oils.

Many herbs noted for their sleep properties should not be used by pregnant and/or nursing women, and the use of inhalers with essential oils is not recommended for those with asthma or other respiratory problems. And of course, as with any outside sleep aid, the potential for dependence, psychological or physical, is present...

67

We strew then opiate flowers
On thy restless pillow,—
They were stript from Orient bowers,
By the Indian billow.
Be thy sleep
Calm and deep,
Like theirs who fell— not ours who weep!
Percy Shelley
Hellas: Song of the Captive Women

You may reach the point where the occasional use of an herbal sleep aid may be indicated. Check not only with your herbalist, **but with your doctor**, before beginning any course of treatment. And don't neglect the other aspects of your sleep program; to place the success of your good night's sleep on an oil you anoint yourself with, a tablet you swallow, or a tea you brew is to ignore your personal responsibility, your **achievement**, in attaining such a restful and satisfying sleep.

Hug

Its powers are amazing, by almost any standards. It can make kids smarter, and adults happier; help cure the sick and heal the wounded. It can make profound positive changes in your mental and physical states. It takes but a second, and costs nothing, to give or receive this healthful gift.

Hug your spouse, your children, your pets. Hug yourself. Give those people you love not just a big hug before bed, but throughout the day. It is a physical act, like sleep, and the more comfortable you are with that, the more you will understand and appreciate your body's needs.

Besides, just knowing how much you love (and are loved in return) will help you to rest easy. And resting easy leads to sleep. See how easy that was?

Hygiene

They were careless people, Tom and Daisy— they smashed up things and creatures and then retreated back into their money or their vast carelessness, or whatever it was that kept them together, and let other people clean up the mess they had made.

F. Scott Fitzgerald
The Great Gatsby, 1925.

Take a good look at your bedroom. The clutter may be contributing to your problem sleep. Clothes on the floor, books and papers on the desk, loose change and jewelry on the dresser or nightstand may be crowding you mentally. And, as we will see coming up next, clutter can be contributing to a number of environmental conditions affecting you physically.

Give your bedroom a thorough cleaning. Pick up. Put away. Open the windows for ventilation. Turn your mattress, and launder the mattress pad. Wash the walls, or if you must, give them a new coat of paint. Shampoo the carpet. Clean your draperies or blinds. Move the furniture to dust or vacuum thoroughly.

A place for everything,
and everything in its place.
Isabella Mary Beeton
The Book of Household Management, 1861.

Organize your drawers and closets to make room for your clothes (and future purchases); it will minimize those busy days when it takes too much time and effort to deal with such crowded spaces. Extend the same thinking to the room as a whole. Sometimes the best way to open up a crowded room is simply to take a piece of furniture *out*; it can make the space seem bigger and simpler: addition by subtraction.

Congratulate yourself when you are finished, whether it takes days, or weeks, or just one afternoon. Survey your new, yet comfortably familiar, surroundings before bed: you are on vacation from clutter, in a room that feels lighter, freer, and larger. You have simplified and beautified your environment, and at minimal cost. As a bonus, by now you could be exhausted! Sleep can only be forthcoming.

> *To live content with small means;*
> *to seek elegance rather than luxury,*
> *and refinement rather than fashion;*
> *to be worthy, not respectable,*
> *and wealthy, not rich;*
> *to study hard, think quietly,*
> *talk gently, act frankly;*
> *to listen to stars and birds,*
> *to babes and sages, with open heart;*
> *to bear all cheerfully, do all bravely,*
> *await occasions, hurry never.*
> *In a word, to let the spiritual,*
> *unbidden and unconscious,*
> *grow up through the common.*
> *This is to be my symphony.*
>
> William Henry Channing

Hypoallergenic

The Food and Drug Administration may have taken exception to some manufacturers' broad use of the term to sell products, but in fact, one of the goals of the above chapter is to make your sleeping area "hypoallergenic". You are minimizing those factors that could trigger sensitivities.

Environmental allergens have been linked to a number of sleep problems, from benign snoring and sleep apneas, to delayed onset and later stage interruptions. There is a good chance, though, that you may have become so accustomed, or the development of such sensitivities may have been so gradual, that you are not even aware of their influence on your sleep.

If you awaken during the night with a runny nose, sneezing, or the awareness that you have shifted to mouth breathing, or if you make it to morning, and customarily awaken with a "stuffy head" that subsides only after a hot shower or being up for a while, you could be allergic to your bedroom! Or at least, to some aspect of your sleep environment.

> *His brother got into bed, and whether he slept*
> *or did not sleep, tossed about like a sick man,*
> *coughed, and when he could not get his throat*
> *clear, mumbled something.*
>> Leo Tolstoy
>> *Anna Karenina*, 1876.

Dust should be the first thing to consider; assuming, that is, your cat Fluffy isn't sharing your pillow at night (allergies to animal dander are among the most common). Your removal efforts should include not just the visible (dust on furniture surfaces, for instance), but the hidden (under the bed or other furniture), the subtly hidden (accumulated on the vents or filters of your heater or air conditioner), and even the microscopic (carpet and dust mites, tiny freeloading roommates), as well.

Other causes of your distress may be equally subtle. For instance, older buildings, with their compromised ventilation, inadequate moisture barrier, and plaster construction, may have molds and mildews growing on or under surfaces in the room.

More recent structures can be the home of allergens, as well. Contemporary building materials (formaldehyde for instance) can trigger sensitivities, even in people that don't consider themselves "allergic". Synthetic carpets and upholstery may *off-gas* for years, and even natural fiber rugs may be bleached or dyed in strong solutions that

71

can cause physical reactions.

Extend the same consideration to your bedclothes. Allergies to wool are common; your blankets or bedspread may use this material, at least in part, in their construction. Even if your **pillow** is hypoallergenic (you may be allergic to down filling and not even know it), the detergent used to launder your pillowcase and sheets may be what's causing your bad reaction.

It could just be that (*just?*) Spring has arrived, in all its glory. Higher pollen counts can make sleep, and life in general, more difficult. A HEPA rated air purifier can help reduce the levels of such airborne allergens.

While they are dealt with in more detail in **diet**, food allergies should at least be mentioned here: they can produce slight, yet often longer lasting symptoms, and commonly go undiagnosed. Do you have more trouble sleeping after eating certain types of food?

Equally subtle may be an allergy to personal products such as perfume, cologne, aftershave, shampoo, hair sprays or styling gels, and hand soaps (or the fragrance used in their manufacture). Though such allergies are common, they can be difficult to trace to their source.

If your environment is in some way toxic to you, your sleep can suffer. If you suspect allergies are contributing to your sleep problems, don't be afraid to take matters into your own hands: clean your sleep environment thoroughly, and remove (if only temporarily) any suspected causes of your reactions. If your sensitivities persist, see your doctor. Once the allergy is identified, most are treatable; generally by removing the source, or, if indicated, through medication.

The breezes were ethereal, and pure,
And crept through half-closed lattices to cure
The languid sick; it cool'd their fever'd sleep,
And soothed them into slumbers full and deep.
John Keats
I stood tip-toe upon a little hill, 1817.

Ideal

Ideals are like stars; you will not succeed in touching them with your hands. But like the seafaring man on the desert of waters, you choose them as your guides, and following them you will reach your destiny.

Carl Schurz
Address at Faneuil Hall, Boston,
April 18,1859.

For many, it is held up as the ideal: you fall asleep, without trouble, at the same time every night; you awaken, rested and refreshed, at your hour of choice.

Few of us have the luxury of the second half of the equation, but let's look critically at the first part as well. Life sometimes seems to be made up more of the exceptions than the rules: to experience it more fully (an admirable undertaking) requires a certain flexibility. Sometimes you are given, or give yourself, the opportunity to enjoy life outside your everyday experiences, so you stay up late. But all too often, it is outside forces (sick children, visiting relatives, noisy neighbors) that interfere with your plans for sleep. If it happens enough, you might even wonder at what point the exception becomes the rule, and your usual sleep can be considered troubled.

Ask yourself what makes an ideal sleep situation *for you*. On what do you base this standard; your own, previous experiences, or things you have read, or heard? Is it based on actual physical needs that are not being met; or do you measure your needs against what you consider to be the norm, or the average? How much more sleep would it take to feel your sleep has improved measurably? What would constitute a major improvement? What is the foremost obstacle to your ideal; and would you remove that obstacle entirely, if it meant a better night's sleep?

Difficult questions, but ones you must ask in order

to establish a foundation for your sleep program. You may find yourself closer to your ideal than you realized, or it may be a more formidable task than you originally thought. Your assessment alone should be cause for neither optimism nor pessimism. But by knowing your ideal, you can not only set goals and measure your progress, you can utilize a variety of behavior modification techniques, such as...

Imagination

It is commonly seen that our cogitations and talk do represent and cause some such thing in our sleep ...such as the mind waking used oftenest to think on.
Cicero, *trans*. Thomas Newton
Scipio's Dream, 54 B.C.

A recent physiological study targeting high school athletes and measuring sports skills improvement produced some rather surprising results: the high school athletes that spent a specified amount of time strictly *imagining* themselves improving their skills showed as much improvement as the group that spent an equal amount of time engaged in actual physical practice. The group showing the most improvement, though, was the one that split the same amount of time doing both, imagining *and* practicing.

While different branches of science have detailed the importance the technique of *visualization* can play in task success, to find that it rivaled physical practice was still unexpected. This finding can bear a profound significance for the sleeper. After all, in sleep, practice *is* performance, and performance practice.

Try thinking about sleep. Not your sleep problems, or the **quality** of it, or the **interruptions** you have been

74

suffering lately, but the actual physical act of you sleeping. You. Sleeping.

Visualize it abstractly, from the third person. Imagine a view of your bedroom as seen from above. When you look down onto the bed, you see someone peacefully sleeping. That someone is you. Observe how you look: eyes closed, with perhaps a hint of a smile, quiet, unmoving. Imagine that this night is like any other, and you, as one of millions enjoying restful sleep, can be found lying there, in that condition, on any given night.

Now, shift your viewpoint to the first person. Imagine what it feels like to be lying in bed, sleeping. You are relaxed. You are content. Your body is motionless; its activity has slowed almost to a stop. Your body is heavy in the bed, so heavy you cannot lift, cannot even feel, your extremities. This is you, sleeping, and this sensation is repeated every night, every time you crawl between the sheets.

Practice such visualization often: beginning when you first wake up, a positive reinforcement of what has just occurred; but other times as well, even when sleep would normally be far from your mind. It needn't take but an instant, and shouldn't interfere with the task at hand.

But keep in mind, it is the quality of the image of you, sleeping peacefully, that holds the power: the vision you see should be completely real, faithful in its portrayal, and utterly familiar. It is, in fact, the way you *are*, asleep. And imagining it can help make it so.

> *Do you comprehend that you are awake? "I do not," the man replies, "for I do not even comprehend when in my sleep I imagine that I am awake." Does this appearance then not differ from the other? "Not at all," he replies.*
>
> Epictetus
> *Discourses*, 101 A.D.

Interruptions

...the soldiers who were his guard, having conceived a spite and hatred against him for some reason, and finding no other way to grieve and afflict him, kept him from sleep, took pains to disturb him when he was disposed to rest, and found out contrivances to keep him continually awake, by which means at length he was utterly worn out, and expired.

Plutarch
Aemilius Paulus, 75 A.D.

Your sleep's been interrupted. Again. Your mate is snoring, your child wants a drink of water, the neighbors are arguing. Invariably, it happens in the middle of a great dream, or on a night when you need your rest the most. But it is not an isolated occurrence; it happens often enough some nights that, like some *aversion therapy*, you don't even *want* to fall back to sleep.

Despite everything, though, you somehow manage to doze off between interruptions. Your body is making the best of a bad situation; while it would prefer a night of uninterrupted slumber, it *can* make do (on a temporary basis, anyway) with such a disrupted sleep pattern. Unless such interruptions are of a regular or prolonged nature, involving multiple phases of your sleep cycle, your deficiency becomes more an issue of sleep **quality** than **quantity**.

One effective way to deter interruptions lies in advance planning. It won't always work, of course; sometimes things happen, and you have to accept, even be glad, for being awakened. But do what you can to reduce the possibilities: keep a glass of water by your child's bed; roll your wife over onto her side if she's **snoring**; shut the window to keep it **quiet**; and, if necessary, use your sleep earplugs or night **mask**.

Be confident in your ability to fall back to sleep. The level of frustration you feel upon each awakening is commonly in inverse relation to your ability to return to sleep easily afterward. The more you learn about sleep and your personal sleep patterns, the more tools you'll have to successfully counter each disturbance.

Above all, don't let an *expectation* of interruption spoil your slumber. You may expect, that if you retire earlier than your spouse, their preparations for bed will interrupt your sleep; or expect that if you've been out late the night before, the trash truck will commence its rounds early the next morning. Since such interruptions are beyond your control (especially any involving your mate's behavior), adjusting your attitude to such disturbances can help diminish their impact, if not their occurrence.

Though outside forces may frustrate you in your search for uninterrupted sleep, don't let the frustration *you create* over such interruptions contribute to your sleeplessness. Sleep between them, and the rest of the world be...well, you know.

Interval

> *But neither does time exist without change; for when the state of our own minds does not change at all, or we have not noticed its changing, we do not realize that time has elapsed, any more than those who are fabled to sleep among the heroes in Sardinia do when they are awakened...*
> Aristotle
> *Physics*, 350 B.C.

If you fall asleep the minute your head hits the pillow, you are *too* tired. You are either not getting enough sleep on a regular basis, or are waiting too long to attempt it. The average, healthy sleeper takes anywhere from 15 to 30 minutes to drop off.

Although I can't emphasize too strongly the part individuality plays in assessing and improving troubled sleep, the above statistic is included for one important reason. If you think something is wrong with you for not falling asleep quickly enough, the only thing wrong may be that your opinion is based upon unrealistic standards. Problem solved.

It is perfectly fine to take half an hour, or even a little longer, to fall asleep at night. Only when it takes substantially longer, on a nightly basis, or you begin to feel the physical effects in your waking hours, should you consider yourself to be "having trouble" falling asleep.

You should calculate how long it's actually taking you; it will be needed if you undertake a sleep **journal** (to come). If using the clock in conjunction with sleep causes anxiety (see **Chronophobia**), develop your ability to gauge time. Practice during the day: note the time, then sit quietly (if at all possible—it's most presleep like— if not, read, water the plants, or perform a similar task). When you think ten minutes have passed, check again. Don't be surprised if you are off in the beginning. As you get more accurate, extend the interval to 20, then 30 minutes.

Your perception of the passage of time can be more than an aid to sleep, it can color your impression of your waking hours, as well. Until recently, my husband never wore a watch. Yet he was never late. He was able to accurately judge what time it was, day or night. Finally, after so many birthdays, anniversaries, and other gift-giving occasions, I ran out of ideas; I broke down and picked out a classic deco style wristwatch for him. He liked the design so much, he even started to wear it, occasionally.

That was the day I stopped wearing mine. And while my watch-weaning was helped by my car's clock, or the one I carried in my purse for lunch hour errand-running, the rest of the time I was left to my own devices. I learned how much of our behavior is based upon time; how we eat, meet, and yes, even sleep, when directed to (and often to our detriment) by the hands of a clock. I developed an appreciation of how subjective time is, and how relative to the task: the sometimes frantic nature of waiting in lines at the bank during lunch hour, or at the race-track window before the flag goes up; the limitlessness of a Little League baseball inning on a summer afternoon.

Knowing how long it is taking you to fall asleep can help you to overcome the anxiety that may be associated with, and contributing to, your sleeplessness. But measure yourself against the norm *only* to indicate how well off you already are, or as a baseline to gauge your personal progress.

Ire

Call for the grandest of all earthly spectacles,
what is that? It is the sun going to his rest.
Call for the grandest of all human sentiments,
what is that? It is that man should forget
his anger before he lies down to sleep.
Thomas De Quincey

Do not go to bed angry. You will toss and turn, stew and fume, when you should be sleeping. Even if you don't outwardly show the more obvious signs of anger: your jaw clenching, your hands tightening into fists; you are reacting physically nonetheless: your heart rate increases, your blood pressure rises, and your mind races. And all that at a time when you need most to be calm, and relaxed, in the dark quiet of night.

Don't lie in bed figuring out what to say next time, or what should have been said, or done, this time. Don't lie in bed, regretting. Do not hate: not the person or thing that "did this to you", not the result of that action, and especially not yourself, for how you feel right now or for "allowing" it to happen.

> *Sweet Pleasing Sleep! Of all the powers the best!*
> *Oh Peace of Mind, Repairer of Decay, whose*
> *Balms renew the Limbs to Labours of the Day;*
> *Care shuns thy soft approach, and sullen flies away.*
> Ovid
> *Metamorphoses*, 8 A.D.

You must free yourself from your anger to manage sleep, if only temporarily. Give your anger the night off. It's *okay*, after all, you're the boss. Vent physically, if you must, but in healthy ways: running, working out, even punching (the heavy bag, that is) and *well before bedtime*. Or escape it mentally, through a movie, music, or a book. If you want to indulge in the rage, the destructive thought processes and debilitating recriminations, do so in the morning, when you are rested and can fully appreciate the stunting effects of such behavior.

While your sleeping dreams can offer respite, and possibly even a solution, lying awake in the dark, with angry thoughts as your companion, will more likely produce only misguided conclusions. Empty yourself of anger, and let sleep fill you instead.

Take a night off from your anger. Just one night, to start. Think of yourself as calm, lucid and self controlled. Your ire is not bottled up, it is not held back; it has evaporated. Then sleep as if you have nothing on your mind. If it happens again the next night, or next week, try it again. Make it a habit, and eventually you will never have to go to bed angry.

And remember that a mind at peace with others is a mind at peace with itself.

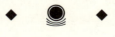

Java

*The government of a nation
is often decided over a cup of coffee,
or the fate of empires changed
by an extra bottle of Johannisberg.*
G.P.R. James
Richelieu, 1829.

Personally, I'm a big coffee drinker. I don't smoke, or drink alcohol to excess (not often anyway), but I love coffee. If I'm reading a book with a scene at the coffee shop, I want a cup. I can see a similar scene in a movie, and unless if I'm sipping coffee *while* I'm watching, I've got to have a cup.

*People who have no weaknesses
are terrible; there is no way
of taking advantage of them.*
Anatole France
The Crime of Sylvestre Bonnard, 1881.

I have learned from experience what may come as no surprise; after all, it is hardly a secret: *all that caffeine can keep you awake at night!* And not just coffee, either, but soda, and tea, and any other beverage with caffeine added.

For some people, it's not a problem if the drinks are consumed before 6 PM., but others have to place the cut-off point in the early afternoon, or even noon, for their last caffeinated beverage. For some, the *cumulative* effects of caffeine can present a problem. You may be one of these, unsuspecting that your three cups of coffee, though taken well before evening, could be playing a part in your nighttime wakefulness.

We're speaking here of caffeinated beverages, but *any* food or drink with stimulative effects has the potential to disturb your slumber. The nicotine in cigarettes (again with significant cumulative potential) has been under increased scrutiny lately, but for others, alcohol (that glass or two of wine, during or after dinner), and even chocolate, can interfere with your sleep.

It may be helpful to figure out *why* you're having that "cuppa joe" during your afternoon break. If you're looking for a boost of energy when your batteries get low, there may be other, better ways: herbal teas and formulas (check for caffeine, just because the label says "herbal" or "natural" doesn't mean caffeine isn't present), a vitamin and mineral regimen, or the natural energy that comes from plain, fresh fruit.

Consider, too, that your body may just be stagnant, not tired: even a few minutes of physical activity can work wonders in restoring vitality. I used to need a caffeinated soda or cup of tea in the evening to have what it took to keep up with my active toddler son. I learned that if I went to the gym more often, and got more exercise, I not only had more energy for play, I looked and *slept* better.

But indulgence *is* often worth the price we pay for it. If keeping score: an after dinner espresso actually has *less* caffeine than a cup of regular drip coffee (despite its flavor and appearance), a cup of black tea less than half that of an espresso, decaf coffee has even less (but usually still some), and an herbal tea need not have any. Whatever you choose as a substitute, it pays to stay away from caffeine, and sleep.

> *One day last week — on Thursday night, to be more exact — I found that I could not sleep, having foolishly taken a cup of strong cafe noir after my dinner. After struggling against it until two in the morning, I felt that it was quite hopeless, so I rose and lit the candle with the intention of continuing a novel I was reading...*
> A. Conan Doyle
> *The Musgrave Ritual*, 1893.

Jet Lag

I certainly cannot undertake to argue that madmen or dreamers think truly, when they imagine...that they can fly, and are flying in their sleep.

Plato
Theaetetus, 360 B.C.

Jet lag is a physical condition that can result from flying to a different time zone. Lethargy, irritability, disorientation, fatigue, and, yes, sleeplessness, are among the symptoms cited most by travelers suffering this malady. Almost all long haul travelers experience it to some degree, and as a rule, the more time zones you cross, the more "lag" you can expect. It is not enough, I guess, to have spent a sleepless night on a red-eye flight; upon arrival you are expected to be awake and alert, even if your body thinks it is the middle of the night. Or you are expected to sleep, though for you it may be eleven o'clock in the morning.

Jet lag is basically a disturbance of your body's internal *circadian rhythm*. This 24 hour cycle, which includes your wake/sleep cycle, can take some time to recalibrate: most estimates of the time needed to regain your equilibrium put it at about one day for each time zone you cross. While there is no cure for jet lag, there are a few steps you can take to create a smoother transition.

Advance planning helps. With the calculated time differential of your destination in mind, adjust your sleep time accordingly (I know, I know, *easy for you to say!*). Try adding or subtracting in 15 or 20 minute per day increments. This amount is gradual enough for most people to handle but significant enough to provide *some* benefits. Try it for a week for a cross country flight; two weeks for a transoceanic one.

83

Besides time differences, some attention to other concerns can help minimize the effects of jet lag. Don't neglect the physical demands that a long flight requires. Don't assume you will sleep on the plane (you probably won't, at least not well), so try to be well rested beforehand. Airplane air is much dryer than you are probably used to, so drink extra fluids; and thinner, so expect alcoholic beverages to have more effect (and aftereffects) than on the ground. Avoid heavy preflight meals, and questionable in-flight ones; you might bring on your own light, nutritious snacks. Stay active on the plane with aisle walks and isometrics, particularly if your time adjustment involves a day and night difference: it can help you stay awake to accommodate a destination's nighttime, or arrive more alert to its daytime hours.

There will be those times you travel so far you aren't even on the same calendar page as when you left. If it is morning, and you haven't had your usual night's sleep, take an extended nap —several hours is okay— as soon as you can. When you awaken, open the curtains to the room, or get outside in the daylight: use the natural **light** to help adjust your body's circadian rhythm to your locale's time. If it's evening, but for you it's morning, attempt sleep only when you start to feel sleepy. When it is morning, again, absorb as much daylight as possible.

There is some evidence to suggest that those travelling in a westward direction suffer less jet lag than those heading east. Children seem more resistant than adults. Similar opinions are offered regarding those who live less structured lives: those on a rigid schedule seem to fare worse than the more adaptable sorts. And one of the few *benefits* of troubled sleep may be found regarding jet lag: irregular sleep patterns can actually help in adjusting to different time zones.

Dietary programs for combatting jet lag exist, though actual claims regarding effectiveness (and evidence of results) are few. Herbal and homeopathic "cures" are sold, particularly those containing *melatonin*, but variables regarding the dosage are critical: incorrect timing or administration can actually make jet lag worse. If you do decide to try these, do so first on a cross-country flight, rather than an around-the-world one; and make certain that critical business meeting isn't scheduled for the day you arrive!

Jet lag can be difficult to overcome. If you are one of those that especially suffers from its effects, preparation can help. If you start by restructuring your sleeping and waking hours beforehand, you will be ahead of the game. If you choose to just wing it, accept its symptoms as an unfortunate aspect of your adventure and go on from there. Good luck, and *bon voyage...*

Journal

I never travel without my diary.
One should always have something
sensational to read on the train.
Oscar Wilde
The Importance of Being Earnest, 1895.

Many people keep one. Late at night, after everyone is asleep, they make their entries: within its pages are both the important events and minutiae of their daily lives. Some call it a diary; I call it a journal. It can be a wonderful tool to learn about yourself, and the world around you. It gives you a chance to not only record, but interpret your life. And as a bedtime, pre-sleep **ritual**, it has a history of thousands of years of leading its contributors nightly from the waking world into the realm of slumber.

A sleep journal, though, is something different. As you travel on the road to good sleep, you will make your way through what seems, at times, a maze: of techniques, information, and experiments. And much like a "trip diary" you would use to record a vacation, your sleep journal will be a record of that journey. Exercising in the morning, rather than the evening? Abstaining from coffee after 3 p.m.? Your sleep journal will help to record such experiments and the results. It will help you learn from your mistakes, remember your successes, and keep you from rewarding any bad habits (sleep related ones, anyway). One benefit of a sleep journal can be seen almost immediately: you will be forced to look critically at your sleep habits, some aspects of which you may not have been aware.

As soon as you can after waking each morning, record that night's sleep. It can be laid out like a spreadsheet, with columns; or in narrative form, like a paragraph of prose. If you opt for the columnar layout, be sure to allow yourself ample room for written details. Record the time you went to bed. Try to gauge, as accurately as possible, the amount of time it took you to fall asleep (as in **Interval**). Note the number of times you were awakened, when they occurred (if known), the reasons for awakening —your opinion, if the cause is not readily apparent— and the amount of time it took you to fall back to sleep. Determine both a sum total for hours slept, and the blocks of time actually spent sleeping.

Write down how you feel, or felt, upon waking: sufficiently rested, or still in need of sleep? Note how you were awakened— to the alarm ringing, some outside noise, or the morning sun streaming through your windows. Glass of wine or two after dinner, espresso, or cigar? Write it down, it you feel it even remotely affected your sleep. Consider, at least, any possible connection.

You are looking for any patterns that develop. The nights you wake up most often may be the nights you retire later. The days you wake up feeling rested may be those with seven hours of uninterrupted sleep. You may find it is not your small child that awakens you as often as your mate's "breathing". You may even come to look at your bedtime differently: were you really in bed, attempting sleep, at eleven, or brushing your teeth at a quarter past, and reading in bed until after midnight?

Your true sleep schedule may surprise you. You may find that you need less sleep than you did when you were younger (a common scenario). You may have considered yourself to be a light sleeper, only to find the opposite is true. Don't be afraid to extrapolate or draw conclusions from this record you are creating.

One thing is for certain: your sleep journal is entirely *of, by,* and *for* **you**. By recording your sleep experiences you are taking an active, hands-on approach to your sleeplessness, and that, ultimately, may be as important as any data your journal may yield.

Juxtaposition

You're lying in bed, after having just found out that your best friend/neighbor/worst enemy/family member just got a new job/house/promotion/pregnant/married, and you're jealous/happy/enraged. Why couldn't it have been you? What if it *had* been you? Why is it always you? Why is it always the other guy?

> *To compare great things with small.*
> *With ruin upon ruin, rout on rout,*
> *confusion worse confounded.*
> John Milton
> *Paradise Lost*, 1667.

Try for one day, or more accurately, one *night*, not to compare yourself to others. Don't hold your accomplishments, achievements, or desires against anyone else's. Chances are, if you haven't been sleeping well lately, you may not give yourself the credit you deserve; all those negative thoughts are at the forefront as you lie there, in the dark, and if you can't even manage something as basic as sleep, well...

In the morning, try this exercise: pretend you exist in a vacuum, unaware of others and how they live their lives. All you know is who you are, where you are, what you are. Now ask yourself: do you need, or want? What? Why? Are these things attainable? If so, what is the best way to get them? Many desires only exist because of others; would you still want something if no one else wanted it?

You may find you don't want material goods, or those trappings that you may have been taught mean success. That's okay, after all, these are *your* goals, not anyone else's. You may readily forsake that luxury car for a chance to go on safari. You may actually be ready to return to school, and study what's always interested you. You may not really want that promotion on your job; you may really want to run your own business.

Even if it turns out you *do* want exactly what everyone else has, at least you are certain of what you want, and why you want it. If your desires stand up to such close inspection, *start working toward achieving them*. Take those steps you decide would most likely result in success, and as you make your way, congratulate yourself on your progress, however slight.

And sleep; you'll need to be rested to pursue your goals.

*It is not fit that men
should be compared
with gods.*
Gaius Valerius Catullus

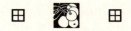

Keepsake

A memento, a reminder of your childhood, a favorite keepsake can help you to sleep. One way to bring about the **comfort** so critical to sleep is by being comforted. While it's recognized as a fairly common technique for helping infants to sleep, we seem to eventually "grow out of it". But when you think about it, is there anything less scary about our adult lives that makes the idea any less practical?

Look for something that evokes pleasant feelings, a happy memory. It's probably something you already have: a photo, stuffed animal, an old toy; anything that makes you feel better about yourself and your surroundings, or that gives you a feeling of warmth and security.

I have a friend who drags Woo Woo with her when she travels. Ragged and torn, this old stuffed dog is with her wherever she goes. How do I know? She has the pictures to prove it. *Woo Woo in New York; Woo Woo in Paris; Woo Woo at the Grand Canyon* ("...oh, look! He's awfully close to the edge in this shot..."). Say what you will, but even when traveling, this woman sleeps like a baby.

While you may not have to go quite that far, do not be afraid to have some cherished keepsake keep you company at night. If you feel especially silly about it, keep it to yourself; that's why it's called a keepsake. So for the *sake* of my friend's reputation, I'll *keep* her anonymous.

> *"Here, touch Woo Woo, you must,*
> *and tell him that you love him.*
> *How 'bout a gander at his trip to Las Vegas...*
> *not right now?*
> *Okay, just let me know when you're ready..."*
> My Anonymous Friend

89

Kimono

Though it sounds exotic, it needn't be; just some sort of wrap or robe, kept by your bed, so that if you have to get up in the middle of the night you will be able to stay warm and covered. This can be especially important if you sleep *au natural*: modesty shouldn't have to be a concern when scrambling around in an emergency.

There are sleep related factors at work here as well. Having to go through a closet in the dark for a wrap just to let the dog out can take you farther from slumber than the simple task would otherwise. And turning on the light risks even more damage to a mental state trying to remain conducive to sleep.

Temperature should be considered, also. The warmth of your bed can be quite a contrast to a chilly house or apartment in the middle of the night; something that keeps you warm and covered can minimize the temperature difference and reduce the "rewarming" period when you do return to bed. As dowdy as they may sometimes seem, slippers perform a similar function.

Of course, if you're having trouble sleeping, the temperature differential *can* be used to your advantage (see **Drop**): a period of lounging about in a state of near (or complete) undress can lower your body temperature, simulating and stimulating sleep; and can make your bed seem especially comforting, warm, and relaxing upon your return. Just make sure your drapes or blinds are drawn, to avoid disturbing *someone else's* troubled sleep.

> *He thought her very tempting in her soft and bright-hued kimono, less refined and delicate than Madame Forestier in her white negligee, but more exciting and spicy...*
> Guy de Maupassant
> *Bel–Ami*, 1885.

Kindness

Anyone who hates kids and dogs
can't be all bad.
W.C. Fields

Think of it as karma (a close *k* relative) without all the accessories, or having to wait a lifetime to check your progress. A feeling of well-being allows a good night's rest. You may eat right, exercise, and have ample full term life insurance, but if you yell at your waiter, poach a parking spot from a stranger, or verbally dress down your subordinates at work you can (dare I say *will?*) have trouble sleeping at night.

A moral disability, no matter how slight, can effect you both physically and emotionally. Be kind, if only for the selfish reason of sleeping better. It may not (initially, anyway) *guarantee* you a better sleep (though it might), but don't stop trying to be a kinder person. It's a lot like quitting smoking: once you've made the effort, it does get easier; and the benefits, though subtle, grow with each passing day.

Knack

The ability to sleep well, at any time and in any
place, I find a great advantage.
Booker T. Washington
Up From Slavery, 1901.

Some people just have a knack for sleep. They fall asleep easily, sleep through the night, and awaken refreshed every day. How do they do it?

First, you may take some comfort in the fact that such people aren't as numerous as you believe: almost everyone, at one time or another, has trouble falling asleep, staying asleep, or getting enough sleep.

But there *are* people that sleep better than others. They have fewer complaints, and derive more of the healthful benefits of sound sleep. What can we learn from them?

We must consider here (again) the part that stress plays. Since it is a notorious enemy of sleep, low-stress lifestyles and occupations, (and low-stress *personalities*) generally sleep better than their higher pressure counterparts. Though you may feel little can be done about your lifestyle or occupation (let alone your personality) your efforts to minimize the cause(s) of stress and reduce its effects through mental and physical exercise can definitely earn you a place among the sleep gifted.

Next is the part genetics plays. It would seem logical to assume that sleep tendencies and preferences develop as you grow, beginning at birth. But some recent sleep research may place the development of sleep traits even earlier: at the moment of conception. Common gene formations have been linked to families sharing certain sleep disorders like *narcolepsy*, or *familial advanced sleep-phase syndrome* (a condition distinguished by a wake-sleep pattern that occurs a full three or four hours earlier than our society's accepted norm). And while it is left to future research to tell us if such genetic predispositions apply to more than just disorders, it is quite conceivable (*sorry*) that heredity may prove to play a large part in determining general sleep habits.

In considering the part that *nature* may play, however, we must also consider *nurture*; in this case, the importance of childhood sleep conditioning. Although, especially as a child, the body will demand sleep to the point of eventually imposing it, the adult raising a child plays an important role in facilitating sleep; they can teach not just the methods for accomplishing it, but the mental attitude most beneficial to achieving it, as well.

Children learn from their parents, through words and action. If the adult caregiver has trouble sleeping, if they are up at all hours, and demonstrate little confidence in their own ability to manage sleep, (let alone instructing others), the child may well come to see problem sleep as, if not the *goal*, at least the *norm*.

Is the Sleep Book engaging in that highly dubious practice of blaming the parents for the ills of the child? Not really; the fact that you're reading this book indicates a willingness to take responsibility for your sleeplessness; and I cannot stress too often in these pages that problem sleep is not a "blame" situation. But it is undeniable that inadequate fundamentals at the earliest levels of *any* endeavor can cause problems later on, even to the point of limiting development. Our mention of any parenting "inadequacies" here is, more than anything, a cautionary one: just by being aware, there is far less chance you will pass on such tendencies, consciously or unconsciously, to your children.

Perhaps the most important thing to keep in mind about people with a "knack" for sleep is the end result: the fact that you may have to work a bit harder, and concentrate more, to find the solution to a problem that others may solve faster and with less effort, should not detract from the fact that you *arrive at the same (correct) answer*. People learn at different rates, even about something as natural as sleep; if your aptitude or background has you studying extra, even having to seek tutoring, in order to graduate, don't despair, or feel you are somehow inadequate. When you finally matriculate to sound, quality sleep, your efforts will have proven more than worth it. And just think, you'll never have to *pull an all-nighter* again.

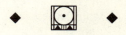

Knot

*"But do you mean to say," I said, "that without
leaving your room you can unravel some knot
which other men can make nothing of, although
they have seen every detail for themselves?"
"Quite so..."*

A. Conan Doyle
A Study in Scarlet, 1887.

Don't think of the answer to your sleep problems as
some gift that, once presented, you will unwrap and open
to discover its wondrous contents. Consider it instead as
a knot that must be undone. You must deconstruct it,
pulling each strand over, around, and through another.
There will be nothing in the center left to discover; instead, each loosened strand will be its own reward.

Remember that each person's sleeplessness has a
cause (or causes). Sometimes you may know it, and just
have to acknowledge it. And even knowing it, sometimes
it can't be helped, like having to care for a sick child or
aging parent. But in many cases the reasons behind a
history of sleeplessness are so complex and intertwined
that it can seem, at times, almost hopeless.

Hence the analogy. Like any knot, pulling on the
loose ends in frustration or confusion will only result in
tightening it. Only by reversing its construction, as a se-
quence, can it be undone. Recognize too, the "hands-on"
nature of the problem: a knot is undone by actually working at it physically; studying and examining the outward
appearance of it usually yields few clues to its solution.

*"So may thy lineage find at last repose,"
I thus adjured him, "as thou solve this knot,
Which now involves my mind."*
Dante (Alighieri)
Inferno, 1321.

Change can be helpful in the initial loosening of the knot; the *push* on the ends that have, to this point, always been *pulled*. Try it in the broadest of terms: stay up late if you've always retired early; try a nap if you've never allowed yourself one. When questioned further, many who claimed they've "tried everything" to sleep actually produce a fairly short history of experiments they've engaged in. Even if such changes in themselves don't bring relief, they may provide a new perspective from which to view your situation.

The big knot of your sleeplessness may be representative of bigger problems. An unhappy marriage, career choice, or frustrating relationships with loved ones, friends, or family commonly manifest themselves in troubled sleep. A mental health professional can help speed the untying, but it still may take months, or years.

Don't equate an immediate inability to reach your **ideal** with failure. Instead take satisfaction in small progresses: even a slight improvement in your sleep can mean more physical energy, and a better mental outlook.

It may help to keep in mind that the convolutions of an especially complex knot may be tied with the same rope as the simplest square knot; and when taken as a series of steps, what appear to be insurmountable problems (sleep included) often have quite manageable solutions.

Courage! All has not failed as yet.
Have patience, craft, for the last knot.
Johann Wolfgang Goethe
Faust, 1808.

Lake

Yes, as everyone knows, meditation and water are wedded forever... It is that image of the ungraspable phantom of life; and this is the key to it all.

Herman Melville
Moby Dick, 1851.

Water is a tremendous soporific. The sound of it. The feel. Conjuring a mental image of water, of lakes and ponds, can lead to the tranquil, relaxed state necessary for sleep. And while we can't dictate the nature of dreams, this liquid realm can provide a casting off point that is serene and peaceful, a favorable condition for exploring the unconscious world.

*Thou driftest gently
down the tides of sleep.*
Henry Wadsworth Longfellow

The sound of water is renowned for inducing sleep. Recordings or simulations of babbling brooks or ocean waves are commonly used to mask ambient noise, replacing the cacophony of the apartment above with the languid shorelap of a beach in Bali and bringing restful relaxation. Usually, that is: some find the sound of waves a constant intrusion to the necessary quiet, and running water...well, the increased need to visit the bathroom during the night *can* interfere with a good night's sleep.

But you don't need audio recordings to derive benefits from the intimate relationship of water to sleep. Wherever you are, whenever you want, you can experience in your mind the calm serenity of a natural lake with a gentle breeze rippling its surface. Imagine the smell of fresh pine, the flash of a fish swimming just below the surface, the call of birds flying overhead. You can experience a vaca-

96

tion, without the hassles of reservations, travel plans, and the cost right now, far from all your worries, lying alone in your bed. Breathe deeply, luxuriate in the mental image of a serene, warm evening canoe ride on a moonlit lake, and sleep.

> *I think of consciousness as a bottomless lake,*
> *whose waters seem transparent, yet into which*
> *we can clearly see but a little way.*
> Charles Sanders Pierce
> *Collected Papers*, 1931-1958.

Light

> *Light the first light of evening,*
> *as in a room in which we rest and,*
> *for small reason, think the world*
> *imagined is the ultimate good.*
> Wallace Stevens
> *Final Soliloquy of the Interior Paramour*, 1950.

We sleep when it is dark, are awake when it is light. Makes sense, doesn't it? In fact, we are biologically programmed to follow this pattern; when we vary from it, problems arise. This relationship of light to our bodies is part of our *circadian rhythm*, the regular pattern of physical responses we demonstrate as living organisms.

Despite the lofty levels we assign ourselves as "advanced" creatures, science has shown we are a lot like other animals, fish, and even plants, in our need for light and the ways it affects us. For instance, the backside of the knee, the *popliteal region*, and other areas of the body far from the eyes, are not only receptive to light (despite the lack of "traditional" mechanisms for such activities, such as the rods and cones of the eyes), they can initiate physical reactions throughout the entire body.

What does this mean for you as a troubled sleeper?

97

First and foremost, a possible reassessment of the light levels in your sleeping area. What you may have considered to be "dark enough" to sleep may be nothing of the sort: while fatigue may be enough to get you *to* sleep, the level of ambient light may be too high to keep you there. Even the light coming from under the door could be enough to awaken you.

Night or "graveyard" shift workers have long understood the necessity for an absolutely dark room to manage sleep during the daylight hours. Even if you do not fall into this category, your blinds or draperies may allow your sleep to be disturbed, or even ended prematurely; by the rising sun, a street light, or even the light of the moon.

> There must be ghosts all over the world. They must be as countless as grains of the sands, it seems to me. And we are all so miserably afraid of the light, all of us.
>
> Henrik Ibsen
> Ghosts, 1881.

Your preparations for sleep may need to take light into account, as well. It may help to dim the room(s) you are spending time in prior to slumber, and avoid brightly lit rooms like the kitchen (make tomorrow's lunch, and grind the coffee for morning, earlier in the evening) immediately before retiring.

If you have trouble waking up, or are a particularly slow starter in the morning, you may be able to use the physiological effects of light to your benefit. While your use of a *dawn simulating* alarm clock may be limited by your bedmate, opening blinds and generally getting as much light into the house as possible may help speed the transition from a sleeping to a waking state.

Lately, clinical sleep research has increasingly focused on the part that light (along with body temperature, another component of our circadian rhythm) plays in "slow starters" and their counterparts, "early risers". As for myself, I became acquainted with such influences first hand. For many years, I had to be at work early in the morning. It was easier on my eyes to leave the lights off, follow shadows to the bathroom, and shower by moonlight. I avoided the light as much as possible. But in those seasons of the year when sunrise more closely followed my rising, I had a different attitude. Sure, my eyes still protested their adjustment, but I felt more awake and alert, if not more "chipper" (after all, it was still ungodly early) at this hour.

Disturbances of our circadian rhythm are an unfortunate by-product of our "modern" lives (after all, why do you think retiring and rising times differed so in the pre-electricity days?); but that doesn't mean we should consider problem sleep a foregone conclusion. Further understanding of the way our bodies respond to light may eventually produce effective therapies beyond those currently targeting *winter induced depression* (and its relative, "cabin fever"), **jet lag** and shift work; it may yield new approaches to problem sleep in general.

At this point, though, things seem to be much more fundamental for the problem sleeper: open your curtains and blinds (and your physical body) to receive as much light as possible during the daylight hour. Close them, as completely as possible, at night. As much as you can, stay in synch with the principle of circadian rhythm, directives your body makes for you (not vice versa). And sleep well.

> *The eyes open to a cry of pulleys,*
> *and spirited from sleep,*
> *the astounded soul hangs for a moment*
> *bodiless and simple*
> *as false dawn.*
> *Outside the open window*
> *the morning air is all awash*
> *with angels.*
> Richard Purdy Wilbur
> *Love Calls Us to the Things of This World*, 1956.

Lullaby

Lullaby. *Lull* a *bye*. As a combination of to "soothe or calm" with "bidding farewell", it is a word particularly suited to its definition (and onomatopoeic, to boot). A lullaby is no more than a "melodic pattern of words or music; usually repetitive in nature". But in the right hands, what power it can have.

> *Her eyes caught the melody and echoed it in radiance: then closed for a moment, as though to hide their secret. When they opened, the mist of a dream had passed across them.*
> Oscar Wilde
> *The Picture of Dorian Gray*, 1891.

Or not. I sang lullabies to my son the first night he was home. It didn't help him to fall asleep when he was one day old, when he was one month old, or when he was one year old. It never worked, and it seemed as if he hardly ever slept. It *did* put my husband to sleep a few times, and it even worked on myself.

I believe now that this was more a reflection of my son's personality and my performance abilities than a diminution of the powers of the lullaby. From Brahms to Gershwin, composers of all persuasions have explored its possibilities; and parents everywhere, every night, improvise them in an effort (sometimes desperate) to get their infants to sleep.

> *Golden slumbers kiss your eyes,*
> *Smiles awake you when you rise,*
> *Sleep, pretty wantons, do not cry,*
> *And I will sing a lullaby.*
> *Rock them, rock them, lullaby.*
> Dekker

We are all infants in our ability to drowse when presented with the right musical stimulus. (As anyone who has either drifted in and out of consciousness at an orchestral performance, or sat near someone who *slept*, snoring, through one, can easily testify.)

One thing to keep in mind (in many ways *the* most important thing), is to take advantage of *all* the benefits that can be realized from creating and performing lullabies. In other words, SING. Sing in the shower, in the car, in public, in the privacy of your home. Don't worry about your talent or ability (or perceived lack thereof); singing can help you to express something that you may not be able to in any other way. Singing can refresh you, revive you, and relax you: not coincidently, many of the same benefits that sleep provides.

If you don't already, start singing. Sing a little each day. Let go. Let it out. Sing of joy, of sorrow, and everything else in between. *Lull* a *bye* to your uneasiness, your self-consciousness, and, with any luck, your sleeplessness.

> *And the lulling melody that had been softer than the wind-harp of Aeolus ...it died little by little away, in murmurs growing lower and lower, until the stream returned, at length, utterly, into the solemnity of its original silence.*
> Edgar Allan Poe
> *Eleonora*, 1842.

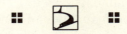

Mantra

One after another those words travelled over my memory, repeating themselves again and again with a wearisome, mechanical reiteration. I was roused from what felt like a trance of many hours— from what was really, no doubt, the pause of a few minutes only— by a voice calling me...

Wilkie Collins
The Moonstone, 1868.

It is a simple concept. You replace those demanding thoughts usually found racing about inside your head with a more basic variety. You assign a word or words to invoke a simpler, more "perfect" image. By repeating these words constantly to yourself (usually verbally), you stifle the more demanding mental processes, and allow your consciousness to enter a state it is normally too harried to consider. In short, you keep your mind focused on the simple to avoid the complex.

In the context of some religions, this usually two to seven syllable group of sounds takes the name of a god, or avatar; and it is believed that repeating it can elevate you to a higher realm of existence. Other belief systems, however, hold that the *repetition* is foremost, and the mantra is merely a first, necessary ingredient for consciousness raising.

In any case, this redirection of thought can be beneficial to both mind and body *and* help to bring about sleep. Which may be reason enough to explore this temporary simplifying of your consciousness, whether your goal is a more godlike state or not. After all, the brain shifts its wave patterns naturally and continuously during sleep; it makes sense, then, to use a similar technique, while awake, to enable its onset.

In selecting your mantra, that word or phrase you will repeat, try to keep it positive and peaceful, or at least

102

benign. And while some groups feel a mental image should accompany the repetition and be an additional focus, others believe that it is the qualities of the sounds themselves that hold the power.

Counting sheep is, of course, a legendary sleep-related variation of a mantra; its repetitive nature induces relaxation, hastening sleep. Therefore, if the religious connotations have kept you from ritual recitation or chanting in the past, you might want to reconsider. Besides, given the increasing popularity of Jewish and Christian mantra based meditation, as well as traditional Middle and Far Eastern religions, spiritual growth (as well as physical benefits) can now fit within more religious frameworks than ever before.

Some time ago, my husband and I got a big kick out of a magazine article based on reader's pet peeves. One woman complained that when her husband got into bed every night he sighed loudly, and proceeded to repeat "bed, bed, bed" over and over again. Sometimes the refrain was broken up with an occasional "ahhhh", then back on to the chorus of "bed, bed, bed". Given the severity of most of the other pet peeves in the article, this man's habit was downright tame; his mantra was certainly as humble and straightforward as they come. But this mental image of the exasperated wife and her chanting husband is still enough to elicit a laugh when either of us picks up this particular mantra after a long and tiring day.

Which may be something to keep in mind: while a mantra is, after all, a personal thing, strictly of and for the person chanting, you should remember to be considerate of any others that may be within earshot. Now, where was I? Oh yes, "bed, bed, bed, ahhhhhhh; bed, bed bed..."

And so to bed.
Samuel Pepys
Diary, Mar. 17, 1661.

Mask

As for poor Leo, after turning restlessly for hours, he had, to my deep thankfulness, at last dropped off into a sleep or stupor, I do not know which, so there was no need to blindfold him.

H. Rider Haggard
She, 1887.

Do you remember the old movies where the spoiled socialite slept wearing a satin mask, and was usually roused only by the butler bringing her (afternoon) breakfast? The pouty insouciance she exhibited upon waking did more than establish her character in the film: it created a prejudice toward this sleep aid that (unfortunately) exists to this day.

The key is darkness: insulating, comforting, sleep providing darkness; a sleep mask (or sleep shade or night shade, as it is also known), is one way to achieve it. If your sleep environment is a place where light cannot be thoroughly or effectively reduced, a sleep mask may be just what you need to make slumber possible.

The frivolous leading lady, despite her character flaws, did demonstrate the utility of the sleep mask: when long nights of revelry (or conversely, when overtime hours of solid, family providing *labor*) turn, too soon, into morning hours, a mask can keep them at bay, and provide extra hours of sleep when daylight would otherwise interfere.

Choose a mask for its comfort as well as its opacity (cute appliques notwithstanding); the elastic band should be wide enough to avoid cutting or pinching for the extended period you will be wearing it, and it should fit snugly, but not tightly enough to cause discomfort. A well designed mask will allow free movement of the eyelids, the best even to the point of allowing the eyes to open completely in their portable darkness.

Oh, and if you *do* try this underrated sleep aid, make sure you have a working alarm clock, or at least a conscientious butler, to be certain you don't end up sleeping the day away.

> *...it lay upon his face, as if to deepen the gloom*
> *of his darksome chamber, and shade him*
> *from the sunshine of eternity.*
> Nathaniel Hawthorne
> *Minister's Black Veil,* 1836.

Memories

> *My eyes still feel the smart of those glad tears*
> *When each grey morn*
> *with slanting beams appears.*
> *Ah does she too, I wonder, think of me*
> *And cherish yet our love's dear memory...*
> Meleager, *trans.* F.A. Wright
> *Remembrance*

Don't let them bring you down. In the middle of the night, the saddest, the strongest, the scariest of them are magnified; the most pleasant, strangely silent. In the darkness our regrets take form; the path they take is the well trod one of your memories. Resist!

As we have discussed, the time you're most vulnerable to the mind's powers is while you're lying, alone with your thoughts, in bed at night. It is almost as if, in anticipation of that period when its dominion over the body is acknowledged, the mind is already warming up, flexing its muscles, exerting its power.

If you are unable to resist, turn insistent memory to your advantage. Choose to relive pleasant experiences: the sound of crunching leaves on a forest stroll, the feel of a sea breeze on your cheeks, the soft touch of a mother's caress; all are available to take you to a realm of relaxation. If memory can't summon these settings, then call on imagination. Just don't get caught up in sentimentality or bitterness, or any similar traps involving value judgements our conscious mind wants to assign, corrupting our memories.

> *I have more memories than if*
> *I were a thousand years old.*
> Charles Baudelaire, 1861.

One reason an infant's sleep is so universally admired (other than by the sleep-deprived parents, that is) is the lack of nagging memories for them to overcome. Their physical needs met, sleep comes easily. Be childlike in your approach to sleep; make your memories, either real *or* imagined, pleasant. And sleep, well... like a baby.

> *A solemn thing it is to me*
> *To look upon a babe that sleeps*
> *Wearing in its spirit-deeps*
> *the undeveloped mystery...*
>
> *Knowing all things by their blooms,*
> *Not their roots, yea, sun and sky*
> *Only by the warmth that comes*
> *Out of each, earth only by*
> *The pleasant hues that o'er it run,*
> *And human love by drops of sweet*
> *White nourishment still hanging round*
> *The little mouth so slumber-bound...*
> Elizabeth Barrett Browning
> *Isobel's Child*, 1838.

Moment

His thought strayed aimlessly... He found it hard to fix his mind on anything at that moment. He longed to forget himself altogether, to forget everything, and then to wake up and begin life anew...

Fyodor Dostoevsky
Crime and Punishment, 1866.

At this point, you are (hopefully) becoming more aware of the thorough connection between your waking state and the **quantity** and **quality** (known collectively as the *efficiency*) of your sleep. Although thus far we have been particularly concerned with behavioral *don'ts*, (as in *don't do that if you want to sleep*), even the *attitudes* we exhibit in our waking lives can influence our sleep.

For one day, tomorrow, try to live life for the moment. When you wake up, no matter how little or badly you slept, be thankful the morning marks the beginning of a new day. You are alive, and that is something to be celebrated; but today, particularly: *for it will be like no other day in your entire life.*

From getting yourself ready, having your morning coffee, making your daily commute, no action will be automatic: today you will appreciate the smell and taste of that hot coffee, the feel of the water on your skin, the motion and the sounds and smells of traffic, in a way unlike any other day. Don't think ahead, of the things you have to do this afternoon. Don't think of the past, even if it walks by in the form of someone you once dated. Don't live in the world of imagination, despite the dreadfully boring presentation at the morning office meeting. Look at everything, no matter how familiar, in a completely different light. See, smell, taste, feel, as if the day were happening to someone new, someone who has never experienced this moment before: you.

...it resembles the ultimate life; for when I am entranced the senses of my rudimental life are in abeyance and I perceive external things directly, ...in the ultimate, unorganized life.
Edgar Allan Poe
Mesmeric Revelation, 1850.

This is not the world of judgements, regrets, and fears you now inhabit; it is simply the world that *is*, all around you.

Will you be able to sustain such an approach to daily life for the full 24 hours? Unless you are a zen master of the highest level, probably not; and even if you are... probably not (which, after all, is one reason why monasteries exist). But try. As your thoughts and behaviors start to stray toward their more familiar territories, call them back. Be vigilant, if just for this one day.

As you lie in your bed that night, stretching and breathing deeply, you will reap the benefits of your achievement. Your thoughts will less likely be of tasks undone, of things said or unsaid; and more likely of the world around you, and the wonder that is daily life. If you are looking for a change, you may have a clearer, even entirely different, understanding of what it is you value, and what it would take to accomplish it. Just by virtue of the tremendous effort it has taken to see the world anew (if only for a day), you may reach a level of fatigue, mental as well as physical, that you have not known before.

And, at that time, you will still know only that moment, that delicious moment of lying in bed without worry, without fear, without distraction. Think only of the comfort, of the tremendous burden of gravity now relieved, of the dark. You will have lived this day for the moment; and at this particular moment you will sleep.

And tomorrow...

Morning

What a singular moment is the first one,
when you have hardly begun to recollect yourself...
Nathaniel Hawthorne
The Haunted Mind, 1835.

It is the single best time for assessments.

Certainly those regarding your sleep. If you are keeping one, this is a good time to make entries in your sleep **journal** or diary. Don't forget to make the qualitative (value) and subjective (emotional) considerations, as well as recording the time(s) and duration of your sleep sessions. And even if you're not writing anything down, when you awaken, at least make a mental note of the **quality** of your sleep and any nighttime factors that may have influenced it.

The first light of day is a good time to dedicate to judgements regarding your life, your career, and your relationships as well. The most significant advantage in establishing this as *the* time for such activities is that you avoid those middle-of-the-night recriminations and regrets, those wee-hour scenarios where you finally give the boss a piece of your mind, and all those other late night, sleep destroying mental wrestling matches.

> *I closed not my eyes that night. My internal being was in a state of insurrection and turmoil; I felt that order would thence arise, but I had no power to produce it...*

We have talked already of minimizing, prior to bedtime, those situations and emotional involvements that could interfere with sleep. The establishment of morning for such activities takes it a step further. You are not avoiding your problems, or avoiding anything, except maybe another sleepless night. Instead, you are dealing with life realistically, dedicating a time for its consideration that will yield most in the way of results.

> *...By degrees after the morning's dawn, sleep came.*
>> Mary Wollstonecraft Shelley
>> *Frankenstein*, 1818.

The light of day has remarkable powers, illuminating not just the physical world, but casting our personal, emotional world in a different light as well. Use it to your advantage: don't be seduced by the apparent calm of night to take on your pressing problems; wait instead for the clarifying light of morning.

Movies

> *"You wake up every morning of your life and you know perfectly well that there's nothing in the world to trouble you. You go through your ordinary little day and at night you sleep your untroubled, ordinary little sleep filled with peaceful, stupid dreams... and I brought you nightmares."*
>> Uncle Charlie in Alfred Hitchcock's
>> *Shadow of a Doubt*, 1943.
>> *(played by the wonderful* Joseph Cotton*)*

There are movies about sleep. There are movies that inspire it. *Sleeping Beauty* is one of the former. Most filmic renditions of Shakespeare fall into the latter category (though several of Orson Welles' versions are exemplary). Some, like *Sleepless in Seattle*, or *Sleeping With The Enemy*, are neither, despite having the physical condition in the title. *Sleepers* is a violent coming-of-age film set in Hell's Kitchen; hardly sleeping material. In Woody Allen's *Sleeper*, the protagonist's affliction is actually a suspended animation resulting from surgical complications. It is hilarious; sleeping through it is close to impossible.

110

Andy Warhol's *Sleep*, though, is surely unsurpassed in either category. Made in 1963, this multi-hour celluloid recording consists entirely of a person (you guessed it) *sleeping*. Despite its potential for inducing same, you probably won't find *Sleep* at your corner video store, even the all-night variety. Pity.

It is common to end up in front of the television when you have trouble sleeping. And a film can be a great deal more appealing than another sitcom rerun. But at the same time, you'll probably want to stay away from "whodunits" or courtroom dramas (you'll want to stick around to find out who, and if they get away with it), genuinely scary movies (even adults have **nightmares**), and war and other action films (for obvious reasons).

I like classic films; the more times I've seen them, the better. With *Top Hat*, I won't be hanging on every line of dialogue or worrying whether they get together by the end, and the Irving Berlin score is tremendous. Nick Charles' wit in *The Thin Man* is as dry as the martinis he mixes, and as entertaining in a half hour snort as an entire "pitcher". As an added attraction, the black and white images of these classics just seem easier on my eyes in a darkened room.

Such films, however, offer far more entertainment than some folks like in their late-night fare; they feel the worst "B" *oater* is preferable to films of quality, and value the eminently forgettable films more highly for their sleep inducing qualities. To them, nothing beats an obtuse European film (just ignore the subtitles), or a Hollywood costumer (particularly if it's set in 19th century England or the time of the American revolution). Of course, the variety of offerings in the early morning hours *is* far different than prime time, and you can see something you've never seen before (or never want to see again).

Ultimately, in movies, as in any other entertainment, it's a matter of personal choice. I feel that if you're awake and watching, you might as well make it something worthwhile. At the same time, if it's *too* good, it's working contrary to your ultimate goal of sleep.

Whatever your inclination, always keep the correct film terminology in mind: a *sleeper* is a trade term for a film that performs better at the box office than expected; a *yawner* is a lethargic or uninspired exercise in cinema. Given the choice, and your need for sleep, you may want to opt for the latter.

> *Don't hate yourself in the morning—*
> *sleep till noon.*
> Daryl F. Zanuck

Mud

> *Life is made up*
> *of marble and mud.*
> Nathaniel Hawthorne
> *The House of the Seven Gables*, 1851.

Have you ever had a mud bath? Neither have I, though magazines sometime picture the upper crust partaking in such exclusive pursuits. I've seen elephants play in the mud, and envied them. Does that count?

When I couldn't fall asleep one sultry evening, I hit upon a mental image that helped almost immediately: I imagined bathing in cool, refreshing...mud. I wallowed in it (there is no other word to describe it, really). It was a liquid world of earthy colors, tactile sensation, and almost weightless support: the nearly perfect medium for creating sleep.

Try it cool, to beat the heat; or as a warm, bubbling mineral mud for the winter season. There's no danger of getting trampled, or even discovered, in the most private jungle you can imagine. Luxuriate in this thick, liquid domain; use its ooze to melt your tensions, and sleep. You won't even get your hands dirty!

"The prince keeps a tortoise carefully enclosed in a chest in his ancestral temple. Now would this tortoise rather be dead and have its remains venerated, or would it rather be alive and wagging its tail in the mud?"
"It would rather be alive... and wagging its tail in the mud".
"Begone!" cried Chuang-tzu. "I too will wag my tail in the mud."

Chuang-tzu
369-286 B.C.

Music

Music has charms to soothe
the savage breast.
William Congreve
The Mourning Bride, 1870.

Wind up crib toys and mobiles introduce children to music at almost the very beginning of life. Its connection with sleep is undeniable. But you would be surprised how many adults with sleep problems have yet to rediscover it, either as a part of their pre-sleep ritual, or as an aid to relaxation, whether it precedes sleep or not. Which is a shame, really. Music is among our greatest achievements as human beings. Its benefits have been proven scientifically; it has few, if any, side effects. And if it can help you sleep, *what's stopping you?*

For some, their prejudices go back to their younger days, when classical music, or worse, *(gasp!)* opera, was shunned because it "put them to sleep". And you are reading this book because...?

But I struck one chord of music
like the sound of a great Amen.
Adelaide Anne Procter
A Lost Chord

You may well feel some trepidation entering a world where Mantovani and Perry Como are deified; if so, some

113

friendly advice: while for some, classical music is...well, a *classic* for relaxation, other types of music may be a better fit for you personally: jazz, instrumental folk, gospel or choir vocals, can all ease you toward sleep. Be adventurous; one person's exciting *Bongo for Modern Swingers* recording is another's ticket to dreamland. Even within the classical world, a Dvorak or Sebelius may be more to your liking than a composer from the pantheon.

Some who try music to help initiate sleep complain that it actually *distracts* them from it. This can be particularly true of vocal music. To those I might suggest *world music*, music from other cultures, performed with unfamiliar instruments, often in unusual time signatures. One advantage to vocals performed in another language is that you can focus on the relaxing attributes of the human voice as an instrument, not on the vocalist's broken heart. The Chinese have a tradition of music composed specifically for inducing sleep; though recordings of Philip Glass compositions may be as effective, and easier to find.

Sleep inducing music may not even be *music*, at least not that performed by humans. Sounds of the rain forest, songbirds, whales, and other natural recordings can certainly qualify.

Don't rule out spoken word recordings or other types of performance, either: audio books can be a way to read yourself to sleep without the eyestrain, and radio shows are television with the addition of imagination. My husband loves to listen to radio dramas of the 1930's and 40's, in a room lit only by the glow of an antique radio's vacuum tubes; a pleasant (if anachronistic) way to meet sleep halfway.

> *Music*
> *heard so deeply*
> *That it is not heard at all,*
> *but you are the music*
> *While the music lasts.*
> T. S. Eliot
> *The Dry Salvages*, 1941.

Naps

Give us, outside sleep,
serenity.
Giorgios Seririades
Mythistorema, 1935.

You're exhausted, and can't keep your eyes open. Or you've got a big date planned for tonight: should you or shouldn't you? Nap beforehand, I mean. Will it keep you from sleeping later tonight; or could it actually help? Experts (as experts are wont to do) are divided on the subject. But it is only recently that research and an increasing dialogue have made napping a truly debatable matter.

Some claim that since we are diurnal creatures, naps are contrary to our development; by disrupting our sleep cycle they will always, or nearly always, hinder our nighttime sleep. Others contend we should sleep when we feel the need to; they cite recent research into cyclical body temperature and our circadian rhythm indicating we *need* naps as living creatures, not just *desire* them out of fatigue or boredom.

Lately there has been another opinion added to the mix: since daytime is the most important time of the day anyway, if a nap can mean a safer, more productive, more enjoyable waking experience, then we should encourage it as a society.

In this country, we are still bound by the Puritan work ethic: we wake up early to go to work, five (or more) days of the week. We get short breaks (or are supposed to, anyway), and, except for an hour (or less) for a midday meal, we work until sunset. The few hours remaining in the day are intended to relax and refresh us; but this is also the time for the traditionally large dinner, family obligations, and cable television. Then it is time to go to bed to rest up for the next day.

You'll notice the lack of time set aside for napping:

if we are particularly tired after lunch, say, we're just expected to go to bed earlier that night. Once past kindergarten, the habit of napping is considered undesirable in our society.

Early to bed and early to rise,
makes a man healthy, wealthy,
and wise.
Benjamin Franklin
Poor Richard's Almanac, 1735.

In many other cultures, the day transpires differently: stores close and business ceases for two to three hours around midday; the people enjoy a rest period that may or may not include a nap. They return to work later in the afternoon, and work until well after dark, eating a later (and generally lighter) dinner, then going to bed. Whether this afternoon period is called a *siesta* or something else, it is common enough to warrant recognition as an acceptable pattern of human behavior.

...and when midday was fairly come, scarcely
a sound was to be heard in the valley— a deep
sleep fell upon all. The luxurious siesta was
hardly ever omitted...
Herman Melville
Typee, 1846.

Some places I have worked have had "nap rooms", a perfectly civilized approach to this very human need. And good business, to boot: there were days I would have called in sick, or left early, if I didn't have a place to close my eyes during my lunch hour. Because often, a short nap is just what is needed to get you through the day safely and effectively: it is, for instance, the most successful technique for dealing with the early morning sleepiness that a long haul trucker (or your airline pilot, for that matter) commonly suffers.

You would be amazed at how much just fifteen min-

116

utes can help. (On the other hand, I have seen plenty of mussed hairdos and cheeks deeply creased by auto interior vinyl, as a nap lasted from morning break through lunch hour. Whoops! "Was anybody looking for me?" they whisper, as they move through the office.)

To decide if napping is right for you, you must first determine if it is even feasible. If it involves putting your head down on your desk, or retreating to your car's back seat at lunchtime, you may not feel comfortable with the idea.

But even if you can nap, should you? *It depends*. If you are tired from lack of nighttime sleep, particularly in that early afternoon period, have access, the time, and the physical environment conducive to it, then try it. *If* a nap doesn't leave you feeling groggy (a common side effect), and *if* it doesn't detrimentally affect your nighttime sleep, then it may be just what you need. But keep it short (no more than 30 minutes), and try to confine it to the early afternoon: the longer it lasts, and the later it occurs, the more likely it will be to disrupt your nighttime sleep cycle.

Try to avoid the *post-work nap*: while it might feel great to get horizontal with your feet up, resist nodding off. Your body may actually interpret this nap as the beginning of real sleep, and everything that occurs subsequently (including awakening and your later nighttime sleep) as a series of confused cycles. And even a brief nap in the evening can delay the onset of sleep.

Remember that naps are primarily for *refreshment*, and can help you **catch up** on sleep, particularly after schedule changes, special situations like traveling, or extended physical or mental labor. They are not designed to replace quality nighttime sleep, only augment it. When you start successfully sleeping, deeply, through the night, or start receiving your **ideal** amount of sleep time, you may see your need for a daytime nap diminish.

For those with small infants (among those most in

117

need of supplemental sleep, at least temporarily) the basic rule still applies: nap when the kids nap. You can never accurately predict, or depend on, when the moment may again present itself. For those of you that work or live with people that *act* like small infants, a nap may be just what you need, too, to recharge the batteries. Just don't let it interfere with, or substitute for, your sound nighttime slumber.

Early to rise and early to bed
makes a male healthy and wealthy
and dead.
James Thurber
Fables for Our Time, 1940.

Narcotics

It astonished me how long the drug took to
act. This, in fact, marked the extent of her
weakness. The time seemed endless until sleep
began to flicker in her eyelids. At last, however,
the narcotic began to manifest its potency; and
she fell into a deep sleep.

Bram Stoker
Dracula, 1897.

There is no shortage of "sleeping pills" on the market, both over-the-counter and by doctor's prescription. Pills to help you fall asleep; pills to help you stay asleep. Whether based completely on natural, herbal ingredients, on modified organic ingredients, or compounded entirely of man-made chemicals in complex formulations, more narcotic sleep aids are sold and consumed every year.

And, if you accept Webster's definition as "a drug that dulls the senses and induces sleep", the field containing sleeping pills becomes even broader, since a *drug* can be anything that "produces a marked change in mental status".

Why, in the context of this book, this sudden interest in semantics? Just this: as a society, we have become increasingly enamored of the "quick fix", especially when it involves our health or our bodies. Many figure that if a good night's sleep can be had just by opening a bottle, (particularly if it's "just" an herbal or natural remedy) why shouldn't we take advantage of it? Especially when it's so readily available.

Certainly, one good reason to look carefully at this practice is *habituation*. (The term is used here to distinguish it from *addiction*, a word so surrounded by negative connotation as to be removed from objective discussion.) Habituation considers the often subtle, yet nearly unavoidable and ultimately profound effects of taking something (in this case a pill, an herb, a concoction) to produce a desired effect (sleep) on a regular basis.

Forget for a moment about *dependence*; think in terms of *conditioned response*: we behave much the same way any intelligent animal does when a reward accompanies a certain behavior. Is this necessarily a bad thing? Not always. In fact, a great deal of the behavior modification the Sleep Book proposes is based on identifying and removing those actions that result in an undesirable response (poor sleep) and replacing them with behaviors that will prove more rewarding.

But the inherent limitations of a bottled **cure** are obvious. For many, sleep becomes impossible without that thing (often artificial) that in their mind "produces" it; without it, they feel they cannot sleep. Also, it is common to need increasing doses to produce the expected benefit. And patients may "challenge" a drug (often successfully) to prove its effectiveness.

Are there times when use of a narcotic is acceptable for bringing about sleep? Of course. In fact, under a doctor's care, the temporary use of sleeping pills may help you to see what a good night's sleep can indeed do for you. To wake up rested and refreshed may help you realize how critical sleep is to both your mental and physical health.

But even if indicated, narcotic sleep aids should be only one component of a comprehensive sleep plan. A competent medical professional should place you under observation, requiring regular medical check-ups and confirmation of your progress. They should analyze your daily habits (and teach you to do the same), put you on a **diet** and **workout** program, (if necessary), and familiarize you with relaxation and stress reduction techniques. They may even have you keep a sleep **journal** to help you *both* keep track of your improvement.

Good luck in your quest for sleep. If you must take sleeping pills, strive to take them infrequently, and very temporarily.

> *Oppressed by the recollection of my various misfortunes, I now swallowed double my usual quantity and soon slept profoundly. But sleep did not afford me respite from thought and misery; my dreams presented a thousand objects that scared me.*
> Mary Wollstonecraft Shelley
> *Frankenstein*, 1818.

Nightmares

Everyone has them once in a while. Sometimes they're just below the surface of your consciousness, waiting for you to get sleepy enough after a slasher film to wreak havoc on your dreams. Other times they dwell deeper, subtly exerting their twisted influence: a strange figure lurking, or pursuing you from dream to dream; someone close to you suddenly in peril. No matter what your parents might have told you, bogeymen *do* exist; they live in our nightmares.

Nightmares can be anything from curiously off-putting to absolutely terrifying. They can certainly interfere with your sleep, even to the point of making it impossible.

For most people (and most nightmares), the expedient way to deal with them is to make them go away. Unfortunately, (especially for the problem sleeper), that means *waking up*. In the case of a nightmare serious enough to awaken you, trust that your mind and body know best.

Sometimes, if the dream has been *that* disturbing, falling back to sleep is either impossible, or ill-advised. If you must, get up. Have a cup of herbal tea. Watch a bit of television, read a page or two of a book. Offer your conscious mind some new stimulus, so that your subconscious will have a chance to regroup, as well.

Nightmares can represent something that is going on in our lives. This may seem obvious. But decidedly less obvious is what the nightmare means, and how it relates to our waking state. Books on **dreams** abound; their quality covers a broad spectrum. While suggested interpretations of common dreams and nightmares may result in *some* self-realization, it is far more realistic to expect only entertainment.

While it is true that nightmares can be a "working out" of waking problems, keep in mind that often, even when progress has been made, or a situation resolved, bad dreams may still rear their ugly head. In referring to our mind as a "slate" on which experience is writ, we should remember that even erased drawings can leave images behind on the chalkboard. Changes in our lives take place not so much in a linear manner as a cyclical one; we grow in fits and starts, and, as animals, operate as much by rhythm as reason. Shouldn't we expect our dreams to operate in the same manner?

On the other hand, recurring bad dreams *have* been linked with increased levels of stress, both mental and physical. Though a nightmare that has you on a speeding treadmill with no off button may be a thinly veiled warning to slow down, dreams involving death, disease, loss, or accidents can also indicate increased levels of stress. Stress reduction techniques may prove beneficial in such cases, both to your physical well being and the overall quality of your sleep.

While confronting your fears (in this case in the form of nightmares) *can* be beneficial, such is not always the case. Coming to terms with them in the daylight can be equally, if not more effective. Additionally, nighttime anxiety about the possibility of a bad dream may also contribute to the frequency and intensity of them. You should feel you are under no obligation to ruminate over a nightmare (or the possibility of one) if it bothers you.

If bad dreams occur often enough, (or with enough intensity) to detrimentally affect your sleep, however, you should take action. If you think you need outside help to resolve the factors contributing to your nightmares, then by all means seek it out. Though nightmares may seem insignificant, even childish, from your waking viewpoint, if the efficiency of your sleep is at stake, then they become very real monsters that must be vanquished.

> *There are few of us who have not sometimes wakened before dawn, either after one of those dreamless nights that make us almost enamoured of death, or one of those nights of horror and misshapen joy, when through the chambers of the brain sweep phantoms more terrible than reality itself...*
> Oscar Wilde
> The Picture of Dorian Gray, 1891.

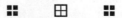

Not Always

Sorry. There will be nights when nothing works. Nothing. You can try every tip, trick, suggestion, or solution you've ever heard, *twice* even, and no go. You just lie there, cursing the coming dawn. Among other things.

To add further to the frustration, you may have a good idea, if not the absolute dead-certain *reason* for your sleeplessness, and may even have taken steps to alleviate it. To no avail. Or, you may have no inkling at all; no connection, however remote, either to your daytime activities or waking mental state, that would have contributed to this (regrettable) situation. Equally frustrating.

You can take some comfort, however small, in the knowledge that it happens to everyone, even "good" sleepers, at one time or another. Don't dwell on it. Keep your eye drops handy for those tired **eyes**, have that extra half cup, if you're a coffee drinker, in the **morning**, and give the new day your best shot. Try again to be cognizant of any activities during the day that may be putting your sound sleep at risk.

That night, try again: a new technique, a different procedure, another approach. If this sleeplessness marks the beginning of a pattern, (or makes apparent a continuing one) consult with your health professional. Just remember that you're on no set time schedule, and don't let an occasional bump in the road stop you in your search for better sleep.

> *Tomorrow too just like today, so without end.*
> *Thus, sir, one's spirits are not always of the best,*
> *but in return one relishes both food and rest.*
> Johann Wolfgang Goethe
> *Faust*, 1808.

Numbering

*...sleep continued to flee him, and he lay awake
with his brain in a state of violent agitation...he
adopted the usual expedients, such as counting
a thousand...to woo the approach of sleep.*
                                   Robert Louis Stevenson
                                   New Arabian Nights, 1882.

Personally, whenever I find myself counting, I know
I'm in for the long haul. It means nothing else is currently working, and I am desperate. Not that some people
don't find this technique successful, which is why the
term "counting sheep" is so often associated with being
awake at night. Or does that make it *un*successful?

Either way, counting isn't a horrible exercise. Just
make sure you are not counting the dots in the acoustic
ceiling tile overhead (do your counting with your eyes
closed), or the alimony payments you have made (keep
the subject matter benign). When I find myself reduced
to counting, I do it backwards, usually from four hundred; it takes a *bit* more concentration than counting forward. Whether it's more boring that way, or less, it seems
to work better for me. Maybe it's more tiring.

Even in counting, there is some room for creativity.
Count by twos. Count in a different language (just don't
berate yourself for never having developed a real facility
for it). Though for some, counting treads dangerously close
to simplemindedness, a chance to engage in a repetitive
mental exercise (see **Mantra**) may be just what you need
to shake your jumble of daily thoughts down to a nice,
relaxed level.

If counting sheep works for you, or if you have never
considered it, then give it a try. This classic remedy (and
cultural icon) may be just the ticket to end your sleepless
nights. For many others, counting, as a precursor to sleep,

is either ineffective or unappealing. If you're one of these, and have no trouble finding other, more productive techniques to combat your sleeplessness, well... you can count your lucky stars.

> *We do not count a man's years*
> *until he has nothing else to count.*
> Ralph Waldo Emerson
> *Society and Solitude (Old Age)*, 1870.

Options

It is what this book is about, really. Sure, the subject matter is sleep, but the primary purpose of these essays is to familiarize you with the idea that the way to sound, productive sleep can be found through any number of solutions.

> *I reflected that man is the veriest slave of custom,*
> *and that many points in the routine of his*
> *existence are deemed essentially important,*
> *which are only so at all by his having rendered*
> *them habitual. It was very certain that I could*
> *not do without sleep...*
> Edgar Allan Poe
> *Hans Phall*, 1835.

In considering your many possible options, it can help to first establish your parameters. If you work during the day, for instance, it's hard to allow that your best time for sleep is from 10 a.m. to 5 p.m. Similarly, if you decide it's important to sleep with your partner, (a critical component of many successful relationships) then you may have to forego sleeping in the hammock out on the veranda. But once the basic ground rules are set, be creative, determined, and above all, optimistic, that you will eventually arrive at the solution to your sleeplessness.

Options can mean compromises. Or not. Your *night*

125

owl spouse has rented the WWII epic *The Longest Day*. As an *early bird*, your options include staying up late to accommodate its viewing, or retiring at your usual hour. You must weigh whether your physical condition the next day is worth the compromise of that (seemingly) *longest night*. (Of course, *Gone With The Wind* may elicit a totally different decision.) Turn such invitations down enough times, though, and other ramifications may be felt. The big picture, including both short and long term affects, and the part other people may play, is something to keep in mind when considering those sleep options available to you.

Family obligations, particularly those involving children, mean additional considerations. You may be up all night by the bedside of your sick child; or up late, **waiting up** for your teenager's early morning entrance. While sleep is important, so is life, particularly when it involves other loved ones. The sleep options viable for you should reflect this.

If being on a strict schedule is the only way you'll get the sleep necessary for your health, then those around you will have to learn to accommodate it. Don't be afraid to call such changes *temporary*, especially if that makes it easier for others to accept at the start; after all, the possibility of flexibility in this strict schedule is a very real one, and it *can* ease them into what are sometimes dramatic lifestyle changes. If you opt to go the strict schedule route, keep the times set aside for your sleep both realistic and accurate: miscalculations can mean frustration not just for you, but for those doing their best to accommodate you, as well.

But even in using the term *strict*, you should never feel trapped or limited, either by your sleep schedule, or the methods and techniques you use to bring it about; I can say with great confidence that there are a world of options available (even given your personal limits) that you have not yet considered.

126

You can, and *should*, try different solutions for sleep. Don't immediately label yourself an insomniac, rush for tranquilizers outside of a comprehensive sleep program, or, perhaps worst of all, throw up your hands in resignation of ever attaining quality sleep. Given sleep's tremendous benefits, it make sense to consider the options available to you, and try any and all that seem to have a good chance of success.

Oranges

I have a room spray made from oranges. Besides claiming to be an all-natural and anti-allergenic air freshener, its label directs you to spray it liberally about the bedroom before bedtime: it promotes itself as an aid to sleep.

Does it work? It *does* seem to make breathing easier, at least temporarily. And there's no denying it makes the room smell nice. I've seen several brands, now, in specialty stores and health food markets. I also have a nighttime face lotion that smells of oranges, and though that's not the reason why I purchased it, it too, claims to have sleep inducing qualities. Granted, it seems every day more products outside the traditional realm of sleep are claiming benefits. And while almost anything that doesn't *hinder* sleep can be promoted as an *aid*, it's good to be skeptical.

But besides aromatherapy, herbal and essential oil therapies have long drawn the connection between the citrus family and sleep: the essential oil neroli, for instance, valued for its sleep inducing properties, is distilled from orange blossoms. There is something, ...well, *slumbery* about the fragrance, if I may coin such a word. Short of planting orange trees outside your window, such

127

preparations may be the easiest way to enjoy the fresh scent of orange blossoms. It may even help you to sleep. It certainly won't hurt.

> *Complacencies of the peignoir,*
> *and late coffee and oranges*
> *in a sunny chair.*
> Wallace Stevens
> *Sunday Morning*, 1923.

Oversleep

> *Hour after hour he lay in his deep sleep. The light of the new day grew and grew in the room, and still he never moved.*
> Wilkie Collins
> *The Moonstone*, 1868.

While it means, in its most literal sense, to "sleep beyond the time for waking", its nuances can extend far beyond the occasional few minutes late for work.

Though it may seem like an oxymoron, oversleeping usually indicates that you are not getting *enough* sleep. You are either not spending enough time sleeping, or not enjoying a sleep of sufficient quality to fully realize all of its benefits. Your body is sleeping past your intended waking in a continuing effort to fill a need; what appears to be a surfeit is actually indicative of a deficiency. Certain hormones necessary for your body's maintenance and growth (in particular, *human growth hormone* [HGH], which promotes the growth, maintenance and repair of muscle tissue) are produced only while sleeping, and even then, only in certain stages of sleep. Miss out on these critical stages, either through insufficient or interrupted sleep, and your body may attempt to reach them anyway, by prolonging your sleep.

How much is enough? To those that contend that even needing an alarm clock to wake up in the morning indicates insufficient sleep, I say, given a choice between having a real life and being in bed (for the sake of a *job*, yet), at 8:30 p.m., I choose the alarm clock.

> *While you here do snoring lie,*
> *Open-eyed Conspiracy*
> *His time doth take;*
> *If of life you keep a care,*
> *Shake off slumber and beware,*
> *Awake, awake.*
> William Shakespeare
> *Cymbeline*, 1610.

A better indication of whether your sleep needs are being met can be found in your condition, both mental and physical, after your alarm awakens you. If you feel disoriented, especially groggy, or physically weak when you first awaken; and particularly if these symptoms hang on after getting up, you're looking at a possible deficiency. Further, if these symptoms result regularly, from your "average" or "usual" night's sleep, then you should critically analyze your sleep habits against accepted tenets of **sleep hygiene**.

While there can be problems that manifest themselves in "too much" sleep, and inordinately long sleep sessions can be the result of, or indicative of, a physical problem, in many cases it is just a result (again) of poor sleep habits. You may have to adjust your sleep program according to your needs.

Often when societal constraints (like a job, or similar regular obligation), are absent, the time allocated for sleep can expand beyond the body's actual needs. The physical and mental symptoms that result can be remarkably similar to a *lack* of sleep: grogginess, lethargy, muscular weakness and fatigue. A vicious cycle often results, with the sleeper sleeping longer in an effort to get more

129

of what they already have too much of. Recent retirees, those recovering from injuries or illness, rest home residents, and others who have had their customary level of physical activity reduced, are particularly susceptible to such a scenario. Even if the only compelling reason is to simply be awake, to the world and its possibilities (and can there be a better reason than that, really?), a regular time to arise may be in order.

> *Ah! my dere love, why doe ye sleepe thus long,*
> *When sweeter were that ye should now awake,*
> *T'awayt the comming of your joyous make...*
> Edmund Spenser
> *Epithalamion*, 1595.

I must stress again the interrelationship of physical health and mental health, and the role that sleep can play in it. "Oversleeping" can be symptomatic of a number of physical and emotional problems, including immune system and nutritional deficiencies, and neurological and chemical disorders. Your body is attempting to maximize that period critical for healing and rejuvenation. Two of the common symptoms of *clinical depression*, for instance, are the increased need or desire for sleep, and the inability to achieve it.

If you are sleeping significantly longer than either the norm or your own previous standards, and particularly if the situation is ongoing, don't delay: see your doctor. Sleep is not one of those situations where some is good so a lot must be better: your **ideal** is, well... *ideal*; direct your efforts toward identifying and attaining it.

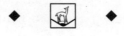

Pain

Pleasure is oft a visitant;
but pain clings cruelly to us.
John Keats
Endymion, 1818.

The pain is so bad you can't sleep. You've tried pain killers. You've tried sleeping pills. You may have tried alcohol, perhaps even in conjunction with pain killers or sleeping pills; a possibly lethal combination. It seems as though no one can relate to your pain, not even the doctors you visit. No one else can feel what you feel. You are frustrated, lonely, and tired; of the pain that has held you in its grip for too long, and the sleeplessness it has brought with it.

Pain can be most generally classified as one of two types: temporary, with either a known, or unknown cause; or chronic, with the same two divisions. In many ways, the scientific study of pain is much like that of sleep: though a part of the human condition since the beginning, only relatively recently has it been given the attention commensurate with the number that suffer from its affects.

Or more accurately, the number of *people* that suffer, since when it involves you, the last thing you're concerned with is numbers and figures and theories, especially those derived from laboratory studies.

Nothing begins, and nothing ends,
That is not paid with moan;
For we are born in other's pain,
And perish in our own.
Francis Thompson
Daisy, 1893.

Like problem sleep, the symptoms of pain can be difficult to accurately describe, its origins hard to ascer-

131

tain. It may not manifest itself in the same way at different times, and may not even be present when medical help is sought. (Don't you just *hate* that?) It can also create a catch-22 situation: by preventing you from enjoying the healing benefits that sleep provides, you are more susceptible to future pain, but more pain means more disturbed sleep. Break this cycle, and the results can be dramatic.

There are many theories regarding the function of pain in humans, both as an individual organism and as part of a species, but most consider it to be primarily a *warning system*: pain is one of your body's ways of telling you *there is something wrong*.

If you are one whose sleep is being compromised by pain and you know its cause, heed the warning and take the steps necessary to relieve it. If you don't know its cause, *find out*; then treat it accordingly. If it is enough to disturb your sleep, it's enough to take seriously; particularly if it is more than just an isolated occurrence.

Unfortunately, chronic pain sufferers often find themselves at a disadvantage: unable to either determine the cause of the pain or to treat it effectively. The future, however, offers hope and encouragement: new advances in diagnostic technologies, pharmaceuticals, and a greater understanding of the part the mind plays in pain (leading to refinements in techniques of biofeedback and meditation, for example), may yet provide you the relief you need to sleep.

> *Bad weather and hard work ...can be borne up against very well, if one only has spirit and health; but there is nothing brings a man down, at such a time, like bodily pain and want of sleep.*
>
> Richard Henry Dana
> *Two Years Before the Mast*, 1840.

132

Pajamas

*"Do you know there are people that
sleep with absolutely nothing on at all?"*
Princess Anne (Audrey Hepburn)
Roman Holiday, 1953.

P.j.'s, nightgowns, flannels, feeties. What do you wear
to sleep in? Like Marilyn Monroe, who reportedly slept
only in her Chanel No. 5, do you sleep similarly,
ah...*unencumbered*, or do you opt for something providing more coverage?

As we have discussed earlier, **comfort** should be a
foremost concern when it comes to sleep; the garments
you wear to bed should meet the same criteria. It is inter-
esting to note that, while fashions have changed tremen-
dously over the past several hundred years, sleepwear
generally has not; while the materials may reflect advances
in technology, the loose-fitting shirt and pant separates,
the oversized nightshirt, or the *union suit* one-piece have
changed little over the centuries.

The oldest sleepwear of all, of course, you were born
with; and wearing nothing at all to sleep in is quite fine,
actually. But if you are the shy type, or live in a place
prone to roommates (or other natural or man-made di-
sasters), then your sleeping attire should be suitable for
getting out of bed in a hurry when your sleep is disturbed.

If you opt for clothing for sleep, (and the majority of
people do) it should reflect the season: brushed fabrics
like flannels and denser knits for winter; combed cottons
and lighter weaves for summer. Flannel has the advantage of only getting softer and more comfortable with each
washing, almost until it's threadbare; at that point it undergoes a miraculous transformation from winter to summer sleepwear. Can you tell that I'm reluctant to part with
a comfortable pair of pajamas?

Since comfort is the key, consider the fit carefully. Are you one of those who don't hesitate to reject everyday clothes because they are uncomfortable, or just don't fit right, but are willing to wear those ill-fitting jammies because your favorite Aunt Claire gave them to you for Christmas? Shouldn't the clothes you wear for that critical last third of your day (spent further wrapped up in additional layers of fabric), get the same consideration?

Figure out what makes you feel secure, comfortable and happy. Experiment with different styles and materials until you find what's most comfortable for you personally. After all, it's for you: people who wouldn't be caught *dead* in a nightshirt may be caught in *bed* wearing one.

And the romance factor of sleepwear? For a couple, it's incurably romantic to share a pair of pajamas, though it's up to the parties involved to decide who gets which half. Sexy negligees? Sure, although many find that which nature provided us to be the sexiest sleepwear of all. If comfort is the goal, the right jammies may be hard to beat; but if eroticism is the idea, well, choose your bed attire accordingly.

> *My uncertainties ended in my taking a way that may make you laugh. I undressed, and put the nightgown on me. You had worn it– and I had another little moment of pleasure in wearing it after you.*
>
> Wilkie Collins
> *The Moonstone*, 1868.

Passion

Cows are my passion.
Charles Dickens
Dombey and Son, 1848.

This is not just about lust and sex, here. Sorry. Seduction and sexual passion are great pastimes, and can lead to a deep, peacefully satisfying sleep.

But passion can be any strong emotion, any "desire that compels" you. And when you're engaged in such passion, sexual relations may indeed be the farthest thing from your mind.

Intellectual passion
drives out sensuality.
Leonardo Da Vinci
The Notebooks, 1508-1518.

Everyone should have a passion, one that needn't have anything to do with a relationship, or even another person. What moves you; drives you? What makes time fly? What is yours and yours alone? What would you do all day, if you could?

You may answer "nothing" and believe it: your job may not be challenging but pays well, the kids are smart enough and well-behaved, and your mate loves you.

But humans are passionate creatures, and in a passionate world, those without it can feel unfulfilled. Passion is the compass for exploration, the required ingredient for any great invention, the emotion behind religion. If you wake up in the middle of the night with a gnawing but indistinct need, it may be better to consider what is *missing* from your life than to count your blessings.

Is there something you love to do, but don't? Something you've always wanted to do? Sometimes finances are a factor (like those flying lessons you've always dreamed of); but often, giving free rein to your dreams can produce creative solutions to such roadblocks, solutions a dispassionate mind could never imagine.

> *Passion, and passion in its profoundest, is not a thing demanding a palatial stage whereon to play its part.*
>
> Herman Melville
> *Billy Budd,* 1924.

Because really, acting on your passion is secondary to possessing and maintaining it, anyway: for every ballroom dancer that needs to be out on the floor three times a week, there is a skiing fanatic that can manage only a couple of days a year on the slopes, or a golfer whose back injury never keeps them from at least *dreaming* about playing St. Andrews. Ultimately, it is what happens in the mind, and in the heart, that makes for passion.

Finding your passion, or rediscovering it, is a part of knowing who you are. The better you know yourself, the better you will sleep at night. Indulge yourself, and your passion, in a healthy, positive way, and you very well could find yourself sleeping better. Good luck, and pleasant dreams; sleeping or otherwise.

> *Nothing is so insufferable to man as to be completely at rest, without passions, without business, without diversion, without study. He then feels his nothingness, his forlornness, his insufficiency, his dependence, his weakness, his emptiness. There will immediately arise from the depth of his heart weariness, gloom, sadness, fretfulness, vexation, despair.*
>
> Blaise Pascal
> *Pensees,* 1660.

Patience

To let the brain work without sufficient material is like racing an engine. It racks itself to pieces. The sea air, sunshine, and patience, Watson– all else will come.

A. Conan Doyle
The Devil's Foot, 1910.

I'm not aware of any studies, and given the number of variables involved, meaningful findings mightn't develop, anyway. But I feel strongly enough about it that I offer it here:

Patient people sleep better.

That's just the way it is. I can tell from looking at that person in front of you in line: they're not constantly checking their watch, tapping their foot, or wiping their brow. They're not rolling their eyes to others in line over the person at the window that's so confused. They are patient. They are calm. I can tell by looking at them that they slept well last night, and will sleep well tonight.

A patient person is willing to wait to fall asleep. They will realize that half an hour (or sometimes more) is not unusual. They know sleep is something worth waiting for, and that building up frustration over not falling immediately to sleep only works against them. An impatient person may already be up after ten minutes, or even if still in bed, may have their eyes open and their dander up, launching into that agitated mode that carries them through the waking day. Their bedtime impatience is symptomatic of a more general condition, an approach to life that emphasizes their *inability* to act over the action itself.

The problem? Such impatience not only effects your mental state, but your *physical* state as well. The expression "don't sweat it" speaks directly to this, as do all those other symptoms (increased heart rate, respiration,

137

and blood pressure, for starters), that accompany such agitation. Of course, this is just the opposite of the physical state you're trying to achieve when you lie down in bed.

The solution? First, don't wait until it's time for bed to practice patience: to find peace at night, seek it during the day. Leave yourself more time to arrive at your destination; don't get worked up over things you cannot change; don't finish other people's sentences, or their crossword puzzles. In short, let your waking behavior mirror the relaxed, confident approach you are currently developing toward sleep. At bedtime, make a relaxing, patient attitude part of your pre-sleep **ritual**, both to prepare you for sleep and to reinforce your improved outlook on life.

Sure, patient people are sometimes frustrating to be around (particularly those *overly* patient sorts), but upon analysis, how much of your frustration is misdirected, intended really for those situations (and which a patient person will no doubt *remind you*) over which you have no **control**?

The patient sleep. Peacefully, calmly, deeply. And if they are awakened, they don't get mad, or frustrated; they wait, quietly and patiently, for sleep's return. So take a page from their book: be okay with falling asleep on *its* terms, not yours, even if it takes a while. After all, you have all night to do it.

> *But I was so tired! And now and again I made a little forlorn complaint to myself that there must often be long delays... Until I dropped, and sleep struck me with its delicious wings.*
> Propertius, trans. J.S. Phillimore

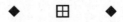

Pillow

She sleeps! on either hand upswells
The gold-fringed pillow lightly pressed;
She sleeps, nor dreams, but ever dwells
A perfect form in perfect rest.
Alfred Tennyson
The Day Dream, 1830.

It's no longer an afterthought, something to fill up a pillowcase. The sleeper of today has an abundance of choices available, from high-tech (the various support system pillows), low-tech (the growing number of alternative, natural filling materials) and almost *no tech* (the eternally popular down feather).

While the health claims regarding any of these various pillows should be taken with a grain of salt (particularly those that *guarantee* sleep), it is true that an uncomfortable pillow *can* interfere with, and even prevent, a sound sleep; and the correct pillow *will* help you to sleep better.

Finding the right pillow for you, however, can be a difficult proposition. Obviously, until you sleep on a pillow (or attempt to, anyway), all claims remain just that, claims. Some of the support system pillows offer a guarantee of satisfaction, something that, given the significantly higher cost, may persuade you to try one. And the especially cost conscious will note that through "knock-offs", and by waiting, sometimes for only a short time, the "latest development" pillows can be had for substantially less than the introductory price.

Do you really need one? A specialty pillow, that is. Products that prey on people's health problems are constantly being introduced, promising a great deal, yet delivering little, if anything, in the way of relief. If you are one of those whose head gets too hot, or too cold, during the night, then the increased circulation that *buckwheat hulls*

139

provide, or the warmth of *down*, may make a purchase worthwhile. Similarly, if you are bothered by neck and shoulder problems, especially during sleep or upon waking, then a *support* pillow can be beneficial. In fact, if your pillow is a concern *at all* when you awaken during the night, consider replacing it.

Because even if you don't have any of the problems the pillow manufacturers are currently targeting, you may be due to treat yourself to a new pillow. Dutifully fulfilling its assigned task every night for years, your pillow may be flatter, lumpier, or generally less comfortable than when it began service. It can improve your sleep to get a new one.

One thing that history (and archeology) has shown us is that, considering what has served as support for a sleeping person's head over the centuries, comfort has been far from foremost: some of the creations of the past were downright, well, *medieval*. And culturally speaking, a comfortable place for the head while sleeping has never been a *universal* requirement.

But practically speaking, if you suspect your pillow is responsible for, or even contributing to, your sleep troubles, replace it. While most of us may not know what constitutes a great pillow, a bad one can make itself known in the worst way. My "Anonymous Friend" (she of *Woo Woo the Dog* fame) takes her own pillow with her on all her trips; though perhaps more sensitive than most of us when it comes to pillows, she feels even spending a single night on a bad pillow is too dear a price to pay. She may be right.

> *...when I placed my head upon my pillow, sleep crept over me; I felt it as it came, and blest the giver of oblivion.*
> Mary Wollstonecraft Shelley
> *Frankenstein*, 1818.

Plans

You can lie in bed for hours making plans; for the weekend, for the holidays, for whatever big day is looming. Or, you can make your plans at some other time and use the time in bed for sleep, thereby helping to guarantee the success of whatever event you are **anticipating**. We have previously discussed the questionable conclusions that may result from late-night considerations (if you're fair skinned, is a week spent sunning on the beaches of Fiji really the best vacation?), but even rational ideas can produce diminishing returns as the opportunity for sleep slides past: to lie in bed at two in the morning making plans to be more organized is a time waster in its own right!

> *Think in the morning.*
> *Act in the noon.*
> *Eat in the evening.*
> *Sleep in the night.*
> William Blake
> *The Marriage of Heaven and Hell*, 1793.

Reduce late night planning sessions by taking care of such activities during the course of the day. Work related scheduling should take place during working hours, and *should be as concrete as possible*. Share some of that responsibility with your co-workers, if possible.

Outside your working environment, make yourself more available to inspiration. Even without a palm PC, you can jot down an idea, or make a note to remind yourself to call someone. Make lists (and revise them as needed), but remember that lists should always be a way to *reduce* stress; if they become a source *of* stress, look to another organizational technique.

You may just need to make more of an effort at *prioritizing*, putting things in order of logic or importance,

141

considered by most to be the critical component of effective planning. With everything else you have going on, lying awake staring at the ceiling over the seating arrangement at your next dinner party may be a waste of your precious time. Decide what's most important, or at least, what's most *urgent*, and your arrangements will be greatly simplified.

Making plans *can* reduce anxiety about the future. It can help with stress, procrastination, fatigue, and myriad other **causes** of sleep problems. And while it cannot remove the possibility of the unexpected (and would you want it to, knowing that the unexpected is a big part of what makes life worth living?), the effectiveness of a comprehensive sleep program is based, in part, on an organized approach to problem solving.

One downside to it, however, is that the conditions most beneficial for effective planning: an extended quiet, relaxed period with a reduced chance of interruptions; usually corresponds to that time just before sleep. Or, more regrettably, that time *intended for* sleep. While it may be fun occasionally to lie in bed and think about your impending party, graduation, or nuptials, for others it can become a behavior pattern that borders on a curse.

Don't let it. Make sure you realize only benefits from your efforts at planning, and make certain that sufficient time for quality sleep is given the importance it deserves. By all means, plan; but save it for when you are well rested. Which, of course, means *after* a good night's sleep.

> *We must plan our civilization*
> *or we must perish.*
> Harold Joseph Lasky
> *Plan or Perish*, 1945.

Practice

Multiplication is vexation,
Division is as bad;
The rule of three doth puzzle me,
And practice drives me mad.
Anonymous
Elizabethan ms., 1570.

Practice. It sounds like work, but it needn't be.

I know, the very word evokes hours spent in some dreary undertaking, whose vague rewards, if they're apparent at all, are far in the future. But if you're reading this book at this point, you know already that sleep is worth the effort; and its actual, tangible benefits are realized not just in that time spent sleeping, but in your waking hours as well.

You must practice in order to become a better sleeper. In many ways, it is like learning an instrument, another language, or any new sport or activity. You may have only glimpses of success mixed in with a lot of frustration. You may have periods where you show scant, if any, progress. And, (for some, the worst insult of all) there are *little kids that can do it without even thinking!* But in other, crucial, ways it is different than these other undertakings.

The first is that you are somehow *expected* to know it. Despite the fact that there are an estimated 50 to 80 million people (in the United States *alone*) suffering from some form of troubled sleep, those without sleep problems often have difficulty relating to those that do. Since their approach to it is essentially unconscious (*sorry*), they rarely have to think about sleep, and consequently have little in the way of practical advice to offer. Which leads us to another difference:

You are expected to teach yourself how to sleep. Unfortunately, this emphasis on autodidactism works against the average person ever finding relief. If you want to learn the violin, or take up golf, it is almost expected you would call on someone already proficient, who would then guide your subsequent education. Medical professionals, however, (especially those of the *sleep specialist* variety), are an underused resource, especially given the number of people in need of their services.

Consider, too, that in sleep, like sex and cooking, practice *is* the performance: while failures are readily apparent, success is often measured in the broadest terms of *acceptability*. While it is assumed that an actor has made all kinds of mistakes during rehearsal for a show, your failure to sleep (the equivalent of forgetting your lines opening night) can make you vulnerable to the repudiation of all your efforts. Don't let it.

In this regard, be aware of your role, too, as the critic of your sleep performance. Strive to be objective, particularly in rendering data for assessments of your sleep. But don't neglect the effect that positive thinking can have on the results. Congratulate yourself on improvement. Give yourself a pep talk when your progress, as it invariably will, flattens out. It is your sleep, and your sleep program. If anyone is allowed to be biased, to positively affect the outcome with partiality, it is you. In fact, I recommend it.

> *Practice is the best of all instructors.*
> Publius Syrus
> *Maxim 439,* First century B.C.

Give yourself the opportunity to learn to sleep. It can take time, but the rewards will be great. Do research: on the subject, and on yourself. Read books about it (you've made a good start). Be aware of accounts and findings of current research that make their way into magazines and newspapers; some of it may relate especially to your situation.

Sometimes a person can't do it on their own. Quite often, actually. You may want to consult with a medical professional, if only to avoid the uncertainties and missteps that can come with any self-improvement program. Especially if your problem sleep is *affecting your health* detrimentally, don't delay: see a medical professional, and if necessary, a sleep specialist.

For the rest of us: practice, practice, practice. It may not get you to Carnegie Hall, but you may enjoy the many benefits that come with a good night's sleep.

> *Practice and thought*
> *might gradually forge*
> *many an art.*
> Publius Vergilius Maro (Virgil)

Problem

You might have already noticed that within these pages the dreaded "I" word is scrupulously avoided; it is called instead *problem* sleep or *troubled* sleep. The reason goes beyond mere euphemism.

There is a great power in words, in their selection and their use. *Problem* emphasizes the need to find a solution, and *troubled* gives a greater emphasis to the temporary nature of the condition.

Insomnia is a clinical term associated with a physical condition for the purpose of identifying its symptoms and treatments. But it is all too often used by those suffering sleeplessness, who have despaired of any change in their condition, and have resigned themselves to it. That's not you. So work on your *problem* sleep, and if you use the "I" word when describing yourself, *knock it off!*

> *The best cure for insomnia is*
> *to get some sleep.*
> W.C. Fields

Progressive Relaxation

I moved, and could not feel my limbs:
I was so light– almost
I thought that I had died in sleep,
And was a bless'ed ghost.
Samuel Taylor Coleridge
Rime of the Ancient Mariner, 1798.

Sometimes a thing is best considered as *a sum of its parts*, rather than as a *whole*. Problem sleep can certainly fit into this category: taken in its entirety, it can seem so formidable as to be insurmountable. However, by breaking it down into its parts, you can more easily identify and correct those aspects of it that are disturbing this natural state of your body.

Relaxation may be considered in a similar way. Although we have already identified it as an important condition for sleep, given its complexity (and perhaps, your personal history) it may seem unattainable in the abstract. "How can you expect me to relax", you may be saying, "with all that's going on in my life!?".

One way to make relaxation manageable is by initiating it through a series of steps. Known variously, but most often as *progressive relaxation*, it is a technique of consciously tightening, then relaxing, individual parts of the body. Focus on the separate areas, and before long your body *as a whole* is ready— for tasks, meditation, or in our case, sleep.

With sleep as your goal, this exercise is best undertaken while lying in bed. You will begin at your feet (more accurately, the toes) and progress until you reach the top of your head. Much like the spiritual/popular song *Dry Bones* ("the knee bone's connected to the thigh bone. The thigh bone's connected to the hip bone..."), each

146

part of the body will bridge with the next.

Lie on your back, assuming a "gingerbread man" pose, with your legs spread slightly and comfortably and arms at your sides, angled away from the trunk. At the aforementioned toes, begin contracting (tightening) the muscles as much as possible. Hold for a count of three, then relax.

Move to the next areas of attention; the ball of the foot, then the arch, the heel. The ankle. The idea is to concentrate, thoroughly and completely, on each specific area. The calf. The knee. Certainly some areas will have little, if any, actual contraction capabilities, but treat them mentally as if they do. The thigh. The hip. Contract. Relax.

Practitioners of this technique seem divided over the preferred mental approach to accompany this exercise. Some say to empty the mind, a bit more with each successive contraction; others say to concentrate exclusively on the contraction/relaxation process, eliciting a kind of mantra effect. In either case, any and all thoughts *disruptive* to the relaxation process should be avoided.

Your breathing should be optimized for relaxation, as well. Use comfortable, measured breaths, and try to avoid the pattern that one would traditionally use with physical activities, such as weight lifting. While this is physical, it should not be work.

It is, in fact, the opposite of work: the emphasis is not on the brief moment of contraction, but on the much longer lasting relaxation phase.

At the end of the progression, make certain you consider the overall, whole body effects of this exercise. Like reading, or listening to music, while you briefly concentrate on the individual notes or words, your emotional response is to the work as a whole.

And don't be afraid, as they say on the labels, to *repeat as needed*. Sweet dreams.

Quality

It is the more subjective of the *Q* brethren, the *yin* to **quantity**'s *yang*. It is based more on your impressions and feelings than on numerical measurements. But it is just as important to consider *how well* you have slept, as it is to measure *how much*.

For most, this consideration occurs almost automatically every **morning**. The general impression of how you feel when you greet the day can tell you a great deal about the quality of your sleep that night. Specific muscular aches and pains (particularly those that diminish after you've been up for a while) may indicate a change is needed in your mattress or **pillow**, for instance. Stuffy head or sinus problems? Consider a more aggressive anti-allergen effort. If you feel like you still need more sleep, an adjustment in your bedtime may be called for.

Such conclusions, of course, are dependent on the fact that your sleep was continuous and undisturbed (as you would duly note in your sleep **journal**).

And if your sleep wasn't interrupted, and you still feel your sleep was compromised somehow?

This is where the assessment becomes more problematic. While it may seem that a new sleep disorder is identified daily, one common characteristic shared by subjects submitting to study is that they didn't derive the expected benefits of sleep (despite allowing enough time for it), *and didn't know why.*

Anyone with a bedmate has most likely heard, at one time or another, "What was the problem with you last night?" Unaware, (if not exactly innocently) you inquire as to what they mean. "All that tossing (or jerking, or grinding your teeth, or various other actions) kept me awake all night." Which, almost invariably, is news to you.

In fact, such increasingly well known disorders as

sleep apnea, *shaking legs* or *shaking limbs* syndrome, and *bruxism*, to name but a few, are more often identified by persons other than those exhibiting the symptoms; persons studying sleepers, or (unfortunately) attempting to sleep next to them. The subjects themselves more often describe vague, nonspecific symptoms, including the almost universal complaint: "I'm still tired when I wake up".

The intent of this chapter is not to convince you that you have some unusual, undiagnosed sleep disorder, but to demonstrate the importance of including a quality judgement in any sleep improvement program you engage in. While the clock may be telling you that your sleep was more than adequate, your body may be saying something altogether different.

Listen to *both*, particularly when you first wake up in the morning. If you continue to have trouble attaining satisfying sleep, and especially if the presence of nagging, nonspecific health problems seems in any way related to that time spent sleeping, consult with a medical professional.

While the amount of time you spend in sleep is an important part of the story, remember that it is just that, *part* of the story. Any sleep program you undergo will prove all the more beneficial by considering quality as well as quantity.

> *It is a new method we have invented for measuring people of quality... We know some susceptible persons who will not put up with being measured —a process which, as I think, wounds the natural dignity of man...*
> Alexandre Dumas
> The Man in the Iron Mask, 1850.

Quantity

Johnson observed, "that a man should take a sufficient quantity of sleep, which Dr. Mead says is between seven and nine hours."
James Boswell
The Life of Samuel Johnson, LL.D., 1791.

It is important to know how much sleep you need in order to feel rested when you awaken. It varies from person to person, but in a most general estimate, the average adult needs between seven and nine hours of sleep per night. Then again, who among us is really "average"?

We all know people that can get by on less than six hours of sleep (and never fail to remind others of it). On the other hand, I have a friend who sleeps more than ten hours a night, takes a nap during the day, and still complains that she is tired. She is training her child to be on the same schedule, and my son wonders why we can never arrange a play date. Inventor, designer, and human theorist Buckminster Fuller experimented with a schedule whereby he slept one half hour every two hours, around the clock; but in his defense, far less was known then about the physiological effects of sleep and the nature of sleep cycles.

You may be unsure of your own optimal sleep time. The demands of daily life and the vagaries of your schedule may have you uncertain of the best time for you to retire at night, or to wake up in the morning.

A common characteristic of most sleep philosophies is the requirement of a standard, fixed bedtime. In this regard, I guess you can consider me the soft-hearted aunt in a family of stern disciplinarians. But a fixed bedtime *is* a necessary component for this information gathering exercise we will use to help determine the quantity of sleep that's best for you.

150

Schedule this exercise when you have a series of days in which you do not have to wake up for anything other than being ready to start your day; a non-traveling vacation, for example.

Begin by establishing a certain time for bed (preferably when you are *tired*); stick with that time for the duration of the experiment. Adjustments will come later; one reason for determining the amount of sleep you need is to help tailor your bed and waking times accordingly.

Don't set the alarm, and let others know they're not to awaken you. Consider the various ways you can be disturbed by outside forces and take appropriate action: turn on the answering machine, keep the curtains closed, wear earplugs and a sleep **mask**, if you must.

Now sleep.

You may be surprised at how early or late you awaken. Or not: the first day or two you will be particularly vulnerable to the force of habit, or the need to **catch up** on your sleep; it will take several days for a pattern to emerge. When you awaken you should feel fully rested; if not, go ahead and indulge that urge to roll over and go back to sleep.

Record the start and finish times for the session, and any **interruptions** to your sleep and their duration, as you will need to factor them in. But withhold any subjective assessments until you have arrived at a representative sleep session; preferably (your schedule permitting) a series of them.

You may be surprised by the result. It is common for people to need less sleep as they get older; your imagined **ideal** may have reflected an earlier need. Or you may find that you are already getting your ideal amount of sleep; this knowledge alone can help resolve concerns resulting from unrealistic expectations.

Your best times for retiring and waking can only be established after knowing the actual quantity of sleep you need. If, even after adjustments, you still feel tired despite receiving the requisite amount of sleep, you should then consider: the **quality** of your sleep, ambient **light** or related environmental factors, **nightmares** and other nighttime emotional disturbances, and other possibilities (including health reasons) for your sleep not being as restful as it should be.

Knowing how much sleep you actually need is a critical benchmark in developing a program to resolve your sleeplessness.

> *...and on the score of sleep, I fully believe that the lives of merchant seamen are shortened by the want of it. ...the crew have a wearied and worn-out appearance. They never sleep longer than four hours at a time, and are seldom called without being really in need of more rest. There is no one thing that a sailor thinks more of as a luxury of life on shore, than a whole night's sleep.*
>
> Richard Henry Dana
> *Two Years Before the Mast,* 1840.

Quiet

We all know someone who can sleep anywhere; at an outdoor concert, in their classroom, in the trenches. Unfortunately, far more of us need it to be quiet in order to fall asleep. While silence may be golden, we live in a world of concrete, metal, and machinery. It can be difficult, especially for the problem sleeper, to find a suitably quiet sleep environment, particularly when sometimes all it takes is the buzz of a refrigerator to keep you awake at night.

You *can* learn to sleep in a disturbing environment. This usually happens out of necessity, lest you are constantly awakened by the *El,* or the nearby highway every

152

time a semi throttles down. You get so fatigued by the continual **interruptions** to your sleep that your body, through a survival mechanism, deigns to sleep through them. And although *learning to sleep through it* is one of the more difficult ways to deal with a noisy situation, it may actually produce the most benefits.

Those inconsistent disturbances that interrupt sleep, though, are both more common and far more difficult to "get used to": the trash trucks that wake you, the neighbor's arguments, police sirens or the occasional car alarm going off. Unfortunately, these examples also indicate how difficult it can be, sometimes, to *remove the source* of the offending noise, another possible approach to dealing with a noisy (sleep disturbing) situation.

The next alternative to combatting such aural intrusions, then, is to *keep them from reaching you*. It can be a challenge. While sound reducing insulation and double paned windows are effective, they are expensive and, let's face it, a lot of work. Intercepting the sound closer to your body may be the answer. Noise reducing earplugs of soft, malleable foam are inexpensive and readily available, and the more effective of them can reduce noise anywhere from 20 to over 30 decibels.

I know: *Earplugs? Seriously?* It might be easier if you think of them as a variation on wrapping the pillow around your head, only a great deal more comfortable and far more conducive to sleep.

Masking the noise is another way to deal with a noisy environment, particularly if your problem lies more in *falling* asleep, than staying asleep. Layering a pleasant sound (water and other natural themes are most common) over the offending one(s) may provide the relief you need, and many players have timers built in, lest the masking sounds become offensive in their own right. Such recordings do have the added advantage of promoting relaxation, another tool proven effective in countering a less than ideal sleep environment.

Quieter and yet more quiet grew the sea, quiet as the soft mist that brooded on her bosom, and covered up her troubling, as the illusive wreaths of sleep brood upon a pain-racked mind, causing it to forget its sorrow.

H. Rider Haggard
She, 1887.

Quilt

What a comforting word, quilt. Pieces of different fabrics, sewn together in a pattern, to make a comforter or coverlet. Quilts have been used to tell the history of an entire group of people. The memories created by a single quilt, handed down within a family, will be of a personal, treasured, nature: a **keepsake** you can wrap yourself up in to sleep.

You can make your own quilt, and start your own tradition, if you've got the time or the inclination. Don't be afraid of it looking homemade: I've even seen them made out of old T-shirts, the ones you just can't part with. Soft, comforting, and a little macho, given those Harley-Davidson and Metallica tees.

Or be more traditional. But be creative; use your imagination to assemble your personal quilt. Because that's what it's all about, isn't it? I mean, otherwise, you'd use just another blanket.

He lay down and pulled the quilt over him... and soon a light, pleasant drowsiness came upon him. With a sense of comfort he nestled his head in the pillow, wrapped more closely about him the soft, wadded quilt... sighed softly and sank into a deep, sound, refreshing sleep.

Fyodor Dostoevsky
Crime and Punishment, 1866.

Read

I gave the matter no further consideration, and at my usual hour retired to bed. Here, having placed a candle upon a reading-stand at the bed-head, and having made an attempt to peruse some pages of the "Omnipresence of the Deity", I unfortunately fell asleep in less than twenty seconds...

Edgar Allan Poe
Angel of the Odd, 1844.

Reading can be a wonderful way to wind down at the end of the day. Something about a book (perhaps it's the lack of loud graphics and insistent advertisements) makes it preferable to a magazine or newspaper for reading in bed. The familiar format, the feel of it in your hands, the look of the words on the page, all help to make bedtime reading a pleasant, relaxing experience.

Read about sleep while lying in bed (you may even be doing that right now). Read some non-fiction, an epic poem, or a philosophical treatise in that time before closing your eyes, and you're expanding your knowledge as well as relaxing your body.

Being read to is certainly among the most pleasant ways to fall asleep. Can you remember that experience from your childhood? How wonderful it was to close your eyes to the sound of a voice, soothing and reassuring, in your ears, leading you and your imagination toward sleep. I've got news for you: it works just as well on adults.

If there's not someone available to read to you at night, you can always rent or buy one. *Books on tape* are available at most libraries, senior centers, and at bookstores everywhere. The quality of the professional actors reading on such tapes can almost make up (*almost*) for not having a parent reading to you. You don't have to worry about *doing* anything; just close your eyes

155

and listen. Recorded lectures (if my college days were any indication) can certainly have the power to summon the sandman. Try Al Gore reading from his own *Earth in the Balance* for a remarkable re-creation.

> *"The deuce!" said he, "there's the match used up. Attention! I can't spend more than a sou a month for my illumination. When we go to bed, we must go to sleep. We haven't time to read the romances of Monsieur Paul de Kock..."*
>
> Victor Hugo
> *Les Miserables*, 1862.

I have a small light that *clips onto* the book I'm reading. In this way, before sleep, or if I awaken at night, I can read in bed without turning on a light and disturbing my husband. A number of booklights are now on the market; some are entirely self-contained, while others involve a smaller lamp assembly connected by wire to a separate power source. Either type is practical not just for home use, but for traveling, as well.

Reading in bed can be a great way to welcome sleep. Just watch the time so you don't stay up past your bedtime, involved in an engrossing page turner. And if you awaken during the night and decide to read, limit it to a short story you can finish, one or two chapters of a book, or, *ahem*, selected passages from this "Bedside Companion".

> *I have read three hours then. Mine eyes are weak;*
> *Fold down the leaf where I have left. To bed.*
> *Take not away the taper, leave it burning;*
> *And if thou canst awake by four o' th' clock,*
> *I prithee call me. Sleep hath seiz'd me wholly.*
>
> William Shakespeare
> *Cymbeline*, 1610.

Relocate

Sometimes you just can't fall asleep in the same spot where you have lain, sleepless, for the last several hours. Or last several nights.

Try a new location. If you sleep alone, try moving to another room. Even the divan (since you haven't actually been *banished* there) is fair game. Just remember to bring your alarm with you if you have to be up at a certain time.

Sometimes you just need a change of scene; sleeping in the same old place can trigger (even unknowingly) the same old habits; the ones that have kept you from sleeping as well as you should. You don't have to check into a motel to realize benefits; just moving to the other side of the bed can seem different enough.

It has been the stuff of comedy for years, the **snoring** mate that drives the other from the bed and into another room; but when things get bad enough, it *can* be what's necessary for a good night's sleep. Of course, if what's keeping you from sleeping is some other, outside disturbance, then even a palatial mansion may not be big enough.

But if all you're looking for is a change of scenery, try it and see what happens; the expenditures are minimal, and you can always return to your regular location if there's no improvement. Assuming, that is, that the family dog has not already claimed it as his own.

> *The Boar could not put me into my usual bedroom, which was engaged... and could only assign me a very indifferent chamber... But I had as sound a sleep in that lodging as in the most superior accommodation the Boar could have given me, and the quality of my dreams was about the same as in the best bedroom.*
> Charles Dickens
> *Great Expectations*, 1853.

157

Responsibilities

Living is a disease
from which sleep gives us relief
eight hours a day.
S.R.N. Chamfort

Sometimes you just have to face your responsibilities. You have to get up early: for work, for school, to care for your children; even though you were up late last night: working a second job, cramming for an exam, caring for a sick child. How are you supposed to get any sleep with all this responsibility?

It may be a small consolation to know that many of us are in a similar situation, with obligations that in various ways keep us from receiving our **ideal** amount of sleep. And I would love to have an easy solution to offer in this chapter, not just for you, but for myself as well. In fact, I sometimes went to bizarre lengths just to avoid acknowledging the connection between responsibilities and sleep.

For years I had to be at work, at my desk, at 7:00 a.m. But the thought of setting the alarm for any time that had a five in it (as in *5 a.m.!*) made me, well... uncomfortable. My mother woke up at 5 a.m. for over forty years to get the kids, my dad, and herself ready for work. To me, five in the morning carried with it just *too* much responsibility.

Realistically, though, I had to be up well before six to get ready, make the commute, and get there on time. So I indulged in an elaborate, if somewhat pathetic, ruse: I set the alarm over forty minutes fast. It felt better on my psyche to see that six-something on the clock, even if it bore no semblance to reality. But then I needed to gauge my morning's progress, so I set the clock in the kitchen, where I would get my morning coffee for the road, somewhere in between. Like tuning a stringed instrument, the

158

rest of the clocks in the house ended up being set *relative*, rather than absolute. House guests often found it disconcerting, to say the least.

What might seem a problem with time (as seen in **Chronophobia**) was instead my problem with responsibility: not a problem in facing or meeting my obligations, but in admitting I had them. When I finally accepted this reality, it didn't matter what seemingly arbitrary number was showing on the clock face. I know when I stay up late I have to get up the next morning, so I must do without my requisite amount of sleep for that day, and strive to go to bed earlier the next night.

Life can be hard (you already know that), and adulthood is a double edged sword: with the increased freedoms come increased responsibilities. The end of childhood certainly didn't mark the end of someone else telling you what you can and can't do. But, as we will see in the upcoming **Rules**, sometimes you can make it easier for yourself by actually *adding* to the restrictions, rather than denying their existence.

> *On a passage, so long as his craft was in any proximity to land, no sleep for Captain Graveling. He took to heart those serious responsibilities not so heavily borne by some shipmasters.*
>
> Herman Melville,
> *Billy Budd*, 1924.

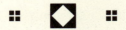

Ritual

*...when I felt assured that all his performances
and rituals must be over, I went to his room
and knocked at the door; but no answer. I tried
to open it, but it was fastened inside.*

Herman Melville
Moby Dick, 1851.

Athletes and entertainers, as a group, are common
practitioners of them. And make no mistake: the regular,
at times even compulsive, pattern of actions they engage
in before a game or performance *can* have an effect on
the outcome. Just don't attribute it strictly to luck.

Instead of good fortune, what these rituals bring with
them is a mental state conducive to success. Rather than
eccentricity, they represent an ongoing process that results in a readiness appropriate to their undertaking. These
certain behaviors tell the mind and body that they are
becoming sufficiently focused for the task at hand.

You can do the same for sleep.

Most people go through a regular behavior each night
before bed; though for many, brushing and flossing and
putting on jammies constitutes the extent of their bedtime ritual. Hardly exotic stuff. For some, checking the
window and door locks provides the reassurance and feeling of **safety** necessary for sleep. For others, performing
small tasks like grinding the coffee, checking their briefcase or ironing a shirt, are more directed toward the next
day.

These regular, even mundane, behaviors all have one
thing in common: they mark both the completion of the
current day, and the beginning of that time for sleep. By
undergoing such tasks, you are letting your mind and
body know that sleep will soon follow.

"Wait a minute", you may be saying, "I put on
jammies and brush and floss (well, sometimes floss, any-

160

way) and I still have trouble falling asleep. What gives?"

While sometimes simply an *awareness* of such behaviors, and the benefits they can provide, is enough to improve your sleep readiness, it may be that your pre-sleep ritual needs to expand, or include some additional techniques. While fifteen minutes of time spent quietly **reading** or listening to classical **music** may provide benefits enough for some, for others specific relaxation exercises, especially those involving stretching, **breathing**, or **progressive relaxation**, may be more in order.

Such ritual activities needn't happen in bed, or even the bedroom; just be wary of including the eleven o'clock news as part of your ritual: while it does effectively mark the end of the day in a regular manner and is of limited duration, the content can be all wrong for your pre-sleep mental state.

Regardless of what form the physical aspects of your pre-sleep ritual take, don't neglect the mental aspects: realize all the opportunities this time provides, not only to relax your mind, but to remind yourself of the deep, satisfying sleep in which you are about to engage. This is not the time for doubts or repudiations; if not a pep talk, at least a well realized mental image (see **Imagination**) of you, sleeping, is in order.

And remind yourself that this is not just *bedtime* coming up, this is *sleep time*; a fine but important distinction. Take it from one who knows.

> *...it was not complete if cold or rainy weather prevented his passing an hour or two in the evening...in his garden before going to sleep. It seemed as if it were a sort of rite with him, to prepare himself for sleep by meditating in the presence of the great spectacle of the starry firmament.*
>
> Victor Hugo
> *Les Miserables*, 1862.

161

Rules

There is a wisdom in this; beyond the rules of physic: a man's own observation, what he finds good of, and what he finds hurt of, is the best physic to preserve health.

Francis Bacon
Essays, 1601.

Almost from the start of life we are exposed to all manner of rules. Simple rules; complex rules. Some rules hard and fast; others more akin to suggestions.

So, given its importance, it is not surprising that among the first rules we become familiar with are those involving sleep. The establishment of *when* a child should sleep, and the preferred method for accomplishing it, are among the first impositions in parenting, with the degree of importance, and enforcement, varying greatly from family to family.

There can be any number of factors behind establishing a bedtime; but there can be a number of benefits as well, including introducing the child to, or familiarizing them with, the concepts of: the **ideal** sleep time and duration, the pre-sleep **ritual**, the need for **patience** regarding the onset of sleep, and teaching oneself to sleep.

As an adult, and particularly as a problem sleeper, you can realize many of these same benefits by setting standards regarding your own sleep. Rules regarding evening activities (especially exercise or caffeinated beverages), a fixed bedtime, and behaviors upon waking during the night, can help you to create a manageable program beneficial to you and your sleep.

For many, establishing such rules for sleep involves them more in the process; but for others, the appeal lies in the fact that it can *remove* them: they no longer have to decide such matters on an individual basis. Some reference books even go so far as to say that the establish-

162

ment of such rules (and adherence to them) is the *most important factor* of your sleep program.

> *...the rules which governed them were sometimes so subtle that mistakes always had and always would be made; it was just this that made it impossible to reduce life to an exact science.*
>
> Samuel Butler
> *The Way of All Flesh*, 1903.

On the other hand, there are few things as depressing as a grown person having to leave a party because it's their bedtime, pass on a Turkish coffee in a romantic interlude because the caffeine would keep them up, or miss a trashy made-for-TV movie because it goes past their appointed hour for retiring.

Yes, establishing guidelines will help you to sleep, especially in the beginning of your personal sleep journey. Yes, the discipline it requires to adhere to rules will help carry you through the inevitable rough spots. But at some point, (preferably *after* you become more adept at sleep) you can and *should* **vary** your routine. Stretching your wings, "pushing the envelope", is part of becoming truly capable at something; sleep should be no exception.

Besides, one of the reasons for seeking better sleep is to have the energy and desire necessary *to enjoy life more*. The more rigid you become, the less you'll enjoy. So work hard at sleeping better, but don't be afraid, eventually, to break a few rules. You'll sleep (and live) all the better for it.

> *They dwell on effects, and modification, without tracing them back to causes; and complicated rules to adjust behaviour are a weak substitute for simple principles.*
>
> Mary Wollstonecraft
> *Vindication of the Rights of Woman*, 1792.

Safety

I was myself somewhat uneasy on the question of our safety during the ensuing night; for I was ignorant of the nature of the extensive country I beheld around me... I accordingly observed to my wife that I would make an endeavour for us all to sleep in the tree that very night.

Johann Wyss
The Swiss Family Robinson, 1813.

You need to feel safe in order to sleep soundly. Secure your dwelling, as much as is possible, against intrusion. Have a phone by the bed for emergencies. Get to know your neighbors (regardless of safety, after all, *they are your neighbors*). Get a dog. Learn self-defense. Think in terms of worst case scenarios.

He looked with terror at the insecurity of his habitation, and went to work to barricade the doors and windows; yet after all his precautions he could not sleep soundly.

Washington Irving
Alhambra, 1832.

All that done, you should now recognize that life is not safe: such guarantees are neither stated nor implied. Do all you can physically to make your dwelling safe, but recognize the existence of a certain element of fear and uncertainty dwelling *within you*: it can only be minimized, not done away with entirely. Nor should you even try; as discussed in **Deep**, it is that part of you that will recognize an unfamiliar noise in the night, sense danger even before it presents itself, and initiate the quick response necessary in an emergency. It is, in many ways, the most important factor in your safety.

But this part of you needs sleep to do its job properly. As a defense mechanism, fatigue can reduce it to com-

164

plete failure in a surprisingly short time. So make all the preparations you must, then sleep soundly, knowing that you are as safe as can reasonably be expected: concern beyond this has the potential to become a danger in its own right.

> *"The purpose you undertake is dangerous"*—
> *Why, that's certain! 'Tis dangerous to take a cold,*
> *to sleep, to drink; but I tell you, my lord fool, out*
> *of this nettle, danger, we pluck this flower, safety.*
> William Shakespeare
> *The First Part of King Henry IV*, 1597-1598.

"Sleep"

You say "Good morning. How are you?" and they launch into their litany of sleep complaints. Or you pick up a newspaper and there's yet another sleep syndrome being identified, or another new medication being touted. It's enough to turn you off to the subject altogether. After all, you have your own sleeplessness to remind you of your failures.

However human this response may be, it is also contrary to the attitude necessary to improve your problem sleep. While the fact that you're reading this book is a good sign (you've avoided the *incurably afflicted* or *utterly exasperated* traps); you can, and could, do more.

When you see the word "Sleep", read what it's about; once strictly the stuff of scientific journals, sleep research now finds its way into popular magazines and newspapers. When others talk about it (and this topic is amazingly popular), listen; a new tip or product is always worth considering. And learn; both for now and for the future.

Don't let your past experiences, or other's failures prejudice you against sleep. Instead, study, analyze, and discuss; within your sleeplessness lies the best way to improve your sleep.

Sleep Hygiene

The one thing he now desired with his whole soul was to... return to ordinary conditions of life and sleep quietly in a room in his own bed. He felt that only in the ordinary conditions of life would he be able to understand himself and all he had seen and felt.

Leo Tolstoy
War and Peace, 1869.

It's altogether different than the earlier chapter, the one that had you cleaning your room. As a branch of science, hygiene is concerned with the conditions or practices conducive to health. *Sleep hygiene*, then, is a term given those variables that constitute healthy sleep practices. You may may be more familiar with them as a list of "Do's and Don't's for Better Sleep", but don't let that discourage you.

The attention paid sleep hygiene can vary wildly: from a virtual unawareness of the subject demonstrated regularly by the sleep satisfied, to the detailed, dogmatic rules of some sleep programs. Your personal connection to sleep hygiene will include not just your sleep practices (including when and how you retire and arise), it may include your sleep history (as recorded in your sleep **journal***)*, as well as those experiments, both failed and successful, intended to improve your sleep.

While sleep hygiene, as a discipline, may be less established than, say, dental hygiene, certain recommendations (like avoiding caffeine and long naps, for instance) have proven effective over time.

Use such established precepts as starting points for your own program. Don't reinvent the wheel. But at the same time, don't be bound by such **rules** as to limit your possible solutions; after all, your situation is indeed *unique*. As a general concept, sleep hygiene is important, but no more so than finding whatever methods, (and there may be many) that will work for you.

> *...hygiene and better taste, consequently a more perfect solution, ...happens when more is obtained by smaller means.*
> Jose Ortega y Gasset
> *Revolt of the Masses*, 1930.

Snoring

> *Then the wolf, having satisfied his hunger, lay down again in the bed, went to sleep, and began to snore loudly.*
> The Brothers Grimm
> *Little Red Riding Hood*, 1812.

It has been the stuff of jokes probably since the beginning of language; yet it is not funny for anyone involved. That rough, guttural rattle can mean trouble, for both the snorer (it has been linked to a number of chronic health problems), and anyone trying to sleep nearby; it is not uncommon for the measured sound levels of snoring to approach that of a busy highway!

> *...requesting pardon for the liberty he was about to take, threw himself upon my body at full length, and falling asleep in an instant, drowned all my guttural ejaculations for relief, in a snore which would have put to blush the roarings of the bull of Phalaris.*
> Edgar Allan Poe
> *Loss of Breath*, 1832.

It is estimated that fully *half* of the adult population snores occasionally, and *one quarter* snore habitually. It is so pervasive a problem that it seems almost a part of the human condition. Yet few people know the causes of it, or that a vast majority of cases can be helped, even cured.

Snoring is basically the obstruction of air movement through the passages at the back of the mouth and nose. Though it can have a number of causes, most snoring occurs for one or more of the following reasons: poor muscle tone in the various muscles of the tongue and throat; excessive length of the soft palate and uvula; excessive tissue bulkiness in the throat; or obstructed nasal passages.

Another common and related, yet potentially more serious, form of nighttime breathing problem is *obstructive sleep apnea*. In this, the sleep of the snorer is interrupted by incidents of completely obstructed breathing; quite literally a stoppage of breath. These interruptions, (and often, accompanying semi-awakenings), can occur for surprisingly long periods and quite frequently during the night.

The effects of apnea are similar to those of any disturbed sleep, only more so: since little of their sleep time is spent in deep sleep, or other necessary phases, apnea sufferers feel especially unrested and sleepy during their waking hours. Besides the increased possibility of daytime accidents and injury, sleep apnea has been linked to chronic conditions like heart disease and high blood pressure. Apnea is considered to be serious if the episodes last more than 10 seconds each and/or occur more than seven times an hour; anyone exhibiting such symptoms should see a physician.

Fortunately, the majority of snorers don't reach this level of sleep disturbance. Unfortunately, even a little snoring can go a long way, and with almost half of all sleepers snoring at least occasionally, well...

> *...he was snoring so loud that it was not easy to convey a noise in at his ears capable of drowning that which issued from his nostrils.*
> Henry Fielding
> *Tom Jones*, 1749.

What can be done for the common (known also as a *primary*, or, in what could be a gross misnomer, *benign*) snorer? Established **sleep hygiene** to help alleviate snoring includes the following recommendations:

Avoid alcoholic beverages and heavy meals within 3 hours of retiring.

Avoid sleeping pills and tranquilizers, muscle relaxants and antihistamines before bed; since overly relaxed muscles in the throat and tongue can contribute to snoring.

Avoid getting overtired. Establishing regular sleep patterns can help here.

Sleep on your side, rather than on your back. Easier said than done, you say? My favorite tip regarding this is to sew a pocket onto the middle of the back of your pajama top, and place a tennis ball in it— just watch how fast you roll over every time you turn onto your back.

Tilt the head of the bed up slightly. This helps too, when suffering from colds and other congestion. The easiest way to manage it is to put spacers —wood or bricks, under the posts at the head of the bed.

Exercise. This cure for any number of physical problems is especially appropriate here, since the lack of muscle tone in the neck and throat area can be a contributing factor to snoring.

These suggestions may prove beneficial, and you may be able to come up with others. Just knowing that snorers (and especially their victims) do not have to suffer needlessly is often a revelation; taking some simple steps toward dealing with it can produce noticeable results with minimal effort.

But I should stress here that anyone whose snoring is detrimentally affecting their health, or others', should seek the advice of a physician. Help is available in various forms; recently developed surgeries mean that far more people with a physical basis for the affliction can be treated. And *everyone* will be thankful for the relief: try as we might, not all of us look upon the snorer, regardless of how much we might love them, as benevolently as we could...

Laugh, and the world laughs with you,
Snore, and you sleep alone.
Anonymous.

Stop

Begin at the beginning... and go on
till you come to the end:
then stop.
Lewis Carroll
Alice's Adventures in Wonderland, 1865.

Stop thinking. Stop worrying. Stop wondering.
Stop. Desist. Cease.
Sleep.

Dear Night!
This world's defeat;
the stop to busy fools;
care's check and curb;
the day of spirits;
my soul's calm retreat
which none disturb!
Henry Vaughan
Silex Scintillans, 1655.

Succumb

Effort supposes resistance.
Charles Sanders Pierce

Admit it. There are times when you are just about to drop off, when for whatever reason, you don't allow it. You rouse yourself. You suddenly remember something you have to write down, or you feel the need to make sure the doors are locked, or your nose itches. And you remain awake.

You have to give up, give in; allow yourself to really *fall* asleep. Don't be afraid to relinquish **control**, to lose consciousness. Sleep is the time to give up the fight, at least temporarily; to regroup, in order to allow even the possibility of future struggles.

> *...awake I try to fight against them, and often enough I do not succumb to them. But in my dreams I always succumb...*
>
> Sigmund Freud
> *The Interpretation of Dreams*, 1900.

Sometimes it's just easier to *forget*. Although in the real world it is considered the lamest of excuses, in sleep it is perfectly acceptable: forget those meetings and obligations, forget your responsibilities, forget everything. Never fear, the real world will provide a wake-up call regarding such matters all too soon. But not right now.

Recognize that sleep is bigger than you. It is more powerful, and more important. If you let it, it can even make you healthier and happier. You *will* succumb eventually, anyway, so why not do it when it's most advantageous for you?

The next time you find yourself in that moment of twilight consciousness, about to drop off, *let go*: succumb. By surrendering, you become the winner.

Suffering

The count fell asleep, but his disturbed slumber
resembled suffering more than repose.
Alexandre Dumas
The Man in the Iron Mask, 1848-50.

Although I may speak in this book of the "art of
sleep", you can rest assured that this is one art you will
never have to suffer for. In fact, you should make things
as comfortable for yourself as you possibly can. Determine what the obstacles to your sleep are, so you can
take whatever steps are necessary to remove them.

Don't suffer in silence. As we have noted in the sec-
tion on **snoring**, among others, problems that are considered to be incurable are often anything but; whether it
is a night guard to keep from grinding your teeth (**bruxism**), a support **pillow** to relieve neck and headaches, or
earplugs to **quiet** noisy neighbors, try to think in terms
of *solutions,* not *suffering.* Talk to your doctor. Read books
and journals. Increase your knowledge and understanding, if only to make available more in the way of solutions.

On a very different, yet highly related meaning of
suffering, avoid that common pitfall of offering sleep up
as penance for whatever wrongs, real or imagined, you
may have committed. Even the **guilt** of having nothing
to feel guilty about is enough for some to say "I haven't
been sleeping well at night", or "I've been up all night
over it". While it may seem a relatively cheap and easy
offering, it is neither: in that curious way life has of operating, just saying something can often make it true. And
anyone with truly troubled sleep can tell you how valu-
able a good night's rest really is.

Such suffering ultimately serves no real purpose.
Sleep well, then spend your energies (guilty or otherwise)
elsewhere.

Technology

So many web sites,
so little time.
Internet junkie's lament

Whether you use the computer for processing data, communicating with friends, or just playing games, it seems like there's never enough time to finish what you've started. While we hear more and more about people becoming addicted to the Internet, even the *use* of a computer brings with it the very real possibility of spending more time on it than you ever intended: you need not be on-line to know how quickly hours can pass while immersed in digital pursuits.

Like nature abhorring a vacuum (or that phenomena that has you filling all your available closet space), the time a computer saves you is not necessarily *extra* time. Throw some disconnects, a crash or two, or an especially elusive data entry into the equation, and watch the hours literally disappear.

The computer is no better
than its program.
Elting Elmore Morison
Men, Machines, and Modern Times, 1966.

It is almost an example of *missing time*, that phenomena of getting on the computer for a simple task (like checking your *e-mail*) and not shutting down until hours later. All too often, the family has gone to bed already; only vaguely can you recall them kissing you goodnight.

The Internet has certainly helped popularize this scenario: since the speed and quality of your Internet connection is usually dependent on the amount of traffic, the best time to go on-line is usually at night, even late at night. The pitfalls inherent in this situation should be obvious by now; add to it the elusive effects of missing

173

time, and you can find yourself sitting at the monitor well into the wee hours. And the popularity of unlimited use plans hasn't helped things a bit.

The solutions to such problems are decidedly low-tech. Budgeting your time is the first step: decide beforehand just how long you should give yourself to complete the task, or how long to play or surf. When you reach that point, *stop*. A timer can tell you when to save and exit; it can even be of the primitive, wind-up variety. Schedule simple tasks like e-mail retrieval for when your time is necessarily limited, like before leaving for work in the morning. Be aware, too, that the morning is often as good a time as late at night for Internet activity; just don't cut your sleep short to log on.

For some, a return to the *per hour* option may be the way to go (though fewer Internet service providers still offer it): to have each minute coming out of their pocket is enough to discourage many. Of course, the truly addicted will spend the time *and* the money; for them professional help may be in order.

Use the computer wisely. It can be great fun, and *is* an amazing tool. But don't be fooled into thinking a faster computer, or a faster Internet connection, will give you more time for yourself, your family, or other activities, including sleep. That will only happen when you decide that those things are more important than the time you spend on the computer.

> *Alienation, if such an overused word still has meaning, is not only the result of social systems, be they capitalist or socialist, but of the very nature of technology: the new means of communication accentuate and strengthen noncommunication.*
> Octavio Paz
> *Claude Levi-Strauss*, 1967.

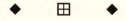

Thanatos

There she met sleep,
the brother of death.
Homer
The Iliad, c. 700 B.C.

It was the god of death to the ancient Greeks, but others, long before and ever since, have explored that connection between the final demise of a human being and that lesser imitation of it that takes place nightly.

For many, it has been held up as the "best way to go": to die in your sleep at night. Even the newspaper obituaries find it worthy of mention when it occurs, both to indicate the sudden unexpected death as well as the merciful end to suffering. And, as something you would not, *could not*, prepare for, for many, that simple prayer recited on retiring summed it up best:

Now I lay me down to sleep,
I pray the Lord my soul to keep.
If I should die before I wake,
I pray the Lord my soul to take.

Were you raised reciting this prayer every night, palms together, elbows on the bed and knees on the floor? Were your eyes closed tightly? Did you add to "watch over Mom and Dad, the baby and the dog", and anything else that meant everything to you? Imagine: to be confronted, on a nightly basis, with the spectre of death, and to have it linked so with sleep. No wonder you are still afraid to fall asleep!

To die– to sleep–
No more; and by a sleep to say we end
The heartache, and the thousand natural shocks
That flesh is heir to. 'Tis a consummation
Devoutly to be wish'd.
William Shakespeare
Hamlet, 1601.

As a small child, I could not get over the fact that just a moment before, my twin brother and I had gone to bed, and now it was morning! Where did that time go, I asked myself; is that what it's like for dead people?

> *Sleep, I have heard say, has only one fault, that it is like death; for between a sleeping man and a dead man there is very little difference.*
> Miguel de Cervantes
> *Don Quixote,* 1615.

It is some justification, I guess, to find out growing up that so many others, in so many different cultures, have also struggled so with this nightly visit to the netherworld, to this land of phantasms and unreality.

But my greater appreciation is reserved for those who, like myself, have come to appreciate that interval of slumber as the *antithesis* of death. It is a time of life, of renewal; not just of the physical body, but of the mental processes and the spiritual self, as well. Waking from a good night's sleep is a rebirth, but a rebirth without death; and each new day is a celebration of life not anew, but continuing, offering unlimited potential for the physical, the mental, and the spiritual being inside us all.

Science has helped remove sleep from that realm of suspicion and superstition; of that we are fortunate. But as long as, during sleep, our bodies continue to physically emulate death, and our mental processes take on those aspects so far removed from our waking lives, the connection between sleep and death will remain. It is not something to fear, but to appreciate.

> *Touching our limbs so gently into slumber,*
> *That Death stands by,*
> *deceived by his own image,*
> *And thinks himself but sleep.*
> John Dryden
> *All for Love,* 1678.

Time

Night and day are not long enough for the accomplishment of their perfection and consummation; and therefore to this end all... ought to arrange the way in which they will spend their time during the whole course of the day...

Plato
Laws, 348 B.C.

I once told my mother that I was too young to spend an entire day checking my watch, counting the hours until "quittin' time". "Oh no," she replied, "that's life. That's what you are supposed to do." But I had so many *other* things that I wanted to do with my life!

When my time, and by extension, my *life*, belonged to my employer, it moved way too slowly; when it was my own, I felt like I was trying to capture lightning in a bottle. And sleep? It seemed I couldn't win.

Given such circumstances, it is tempting to burn the midnight oil; to stay up late or even all night for the chance to get some work done, enjoy a hobby, or just have some quiet time for yourself. Granted, the need to pull an occasional all-nighter to study for an exam, or ready a presentation for a meeting, is one thing. But to find yourself doing housework in the middle of the night, just to get it done, well, there's *got* to be a better way.

For me the answer was to get up earlier. Of course, given the concept of **ideal** sleep time, it meant I would go to bed earlier; but for me the trade-off worked. The extra hour in the morning was a time in which I could accomplish a great deal: if I were so inclined, I could study, and **write**; but I could also relax, think, or just enjoy a cup of coffee and the morning paper, undisturbed. My hours spent at work hadn't changed, but my *perception* of them had: those hours spent at work,

177

away from my *real* life, I now considered to be the interruption (albeit an extended one); I had begun the day on my own terms and would return to it the first chance I could.

Managing your time is tough, and the subject of many books in its own right. My foremost concern here is that you don't shortchange your sleep in an effort to accomplish what you could not in your waking hours. So if the advice I offer here: to *use your time wisely*, and *work smarter, rather than harder*, seems prosaic, it is with the express purpose of helping you *preserve that time for sleep*.

Part of being more efficient on the job is being at your best, physically and mentally. If you are tired, your production, as well as your attitude, will suffer. Once you have determined just how much sleep you need (through your activites in **Quantity**) you can plan your days with the goal of keeping that time required for sleep inviolable. While exceptions are unavoidable (in fact, the variety they provide can sometimes be welcome), your efforts at time management can make sacrificing your sleep no longer necessary.

So in offering this final old efficiency chestnut: *manage your time, don't let it manage you*; I will add that, given the opportunity, time will invariably select that period to fill which is completely devoid of appointments and responsibilities: your sleep time. Don't let it. With renewed energy and spirit, you can take on the world; without it, chances are good you'll always be running behind.

> *Finding nothing in either to induce a change of plan, he lay down, and prepared to catch a few hours' sleep, that the morrow might find him equal to its exigencies.*
> James Fenimore Cooper
> *The Deerslayer*, 1841.

Tomorrow

Out of the shadows of night,
The world rolls into light;
It is daybreak everywhere.
Henry Wadsworth Longfellow
The Bells of San Blas, 1882.

You tried everything. Or, you didn't try anything. But whether it was by choice or not, you were awake all night. And as morning nears, and you prepare to meet those obligations of the waking world, you are *very* tired.

For your own, and others' sake, don't use your lack of sleep as an excuse to be cranky or rude. It helps nothing to direct those raw emotions resulting from your sleeplessness toward others.

Try to make the best of the new day. It is natural, after such a night, to find yourself irritable and distracted, and unable to concentrate for extended periods. Do the best you can, but start by making an honest assessment of your capabilities. Scores of deaths and millions of dollars of costs are attributed every year to workers falling asleep on the job; above all, don't contribute to this unfortunate statistic. Remember that you put not only yourself, but others, in danger by operating machinery or undertaking similar tasks in such a diminished capacity.

Be ready to put coping mechanisms into play; devote some of your depleted energies into making things as easy on yourself as possible, or at least, as easy as is *practical*. Cancel meetings, if you must, especially if you think your compromised condition will put you at a disadvantage. Avoid arguments and disagreements: if you are not at your best, at least avoid being seen at your worst.

Try to learn from the night before, to figure out what you can do to help tonight's sleep. Analyze your activities of the previous day, and consider what part they may have played in your sleepless night.

> *"Very well, very well," said the workman, in good English, "return and tell the king that if he sleeps badly tonight, he will sleep better tomorrow night."*
> Alexandre Dumas
Twenty Years After, 1845.

Don't write off the entire day after a particularly bad night. Do the best you can. Take it easy, and go easy on yourself: if the most noteworthy achievement of the day is that you make it to its conclusion with good humor and patience, congratulations; for that alone is no mean feat!

Tragedy

> *Whether we sleep or wake*
> *the vast machinery of the universe*
> *still goes on.*
> Thomas Paine
> *The Age of Reason*, 1794-96.

You've been blindsided. From out of nowhere, a ton of bricks falls on you: you're struck so hard you're spinning, and when you finally stop, you don't know where you are or even how it happened.

Tragedy. It is the stuff of literature, plays, art, and music. And, unfortunately, life. When it strikes, going to bed can mean a lump in your throat so thick you can't swallow, and a heart that aches even more than your head: you feel mentally, physically, and emotionally drained.

Hopefully it never happens to you. But few, if any, of us are immune: even if you manage somehow to avoid it personally, you can still suffer its effects just by being a member of a larger group, the society of mankind.

When it happened in our family I felt firsthand the ways it can affect sleep: the more we cried, the less we slept; the less we slept, the more we cried. At night, in the darkness, you both welcome the relief (however temporary) that sleep can bring and resist it: the surrender that sleep entails only seemed to emphasize how tenuous, even imaginary, our influence really is over this thing called life.

> Gradually, he fell into that deep tranquil sleep
> which ease from recent suffering alone imparts;
> that calm and peaceful rest which it is pain to
> wake from.
>
> Charles Dickens
> Oliver Twist, 1838.

Remember that there is help, both from trained professionals and those people we surround ourselves with; and it is in tragedy that we come to know best those that mean the most to us. Recognize that you may need to see your doctor for a closely monitored (temporary) prescription to help you sleep. A therapist, or group that has shared a similar pain, can also help bring you the comfort necessary to return to your normal routine.

Expect that it will take time, and that the sadness will be with you, in some form or another, always. Grant yourself the time you need to be alone, for ultimately it is *you* that will have to deal with an existence that allows such tragedy. But surround yourself with friends and loved ones, as well: it is a rare burden that cannot be lessened by sharing it with others.

Sleep may seem the most mundane of activities in this time of upheaval, but you need it, physically as well as emotionally, more than ever. This need is not a weakness, but is as natural and necessary as any we

181

may come to know in our all-too-limited time here.

"Hey, don't worry about me, I'll
be seeing you this summer in L.A.!"
David
In loving memory.

Try

It was the middle of a night like countless others. After awakening for whatever reason, I lay there, as I had so many other times before, staring up at the ceiling. Thinking. I wasn't even trying to sleep; if I didn't have to be up in just a few hours to get ready for work, it would have been a good time to be alone with my thoughts.

It was a scene that had been played out on numerous other occasions, but this time there were some important differences.

First and foremost was that I wasn't stressing over the fact that I was awake. My continuing efforts at improving my sleep had at least brought me to a point where I wasn't mortified to find myself awake at 3:00 am. I was confident that sleep would either occur again of its own accord, or I would be able to induce it, if I only tried.

Which is what happened. Oh sure, there were a few little sidetracks (mentally dwelling a bit too long on the nuances of the Joan Crawford movie we had seen that night, or what I was to wear to work in the morning, for instance), but basically, when I *tried* to fall asleep, really made a conscious effort, I was able to manage it.

Some hidden process was started in you by the
effort, which went on after the effort ceased, and
made the result come as if it came spontaneously.
William James
The Varieties of Religious Experience, 1902.

That night, I learned several lessons.

The first lesson was to avoid that initial *negative* reaction upon waking. While it might seem an entirely appropriate response, it can set up an attitude of defeat and despair that can be difficult, even impossible, to overcome. Yes, you are awake (again), but no amount of self-loathing will change that; only falling back to sleep will. Waking up in the middle of the night is not the end of the world, only an **interruption** of your rest.

The other important concept I came away with that night was a new understanding of the importance of *trying*. Be certain that you're indeed *making the effort* to fall asleep, not just using your wakefulness as an *excuse not to*. Be honest with yourself and objective about your situation, and avoid lamenting your inability to sleep. Far more benefits can be found by saying "What else can I be doing?" than "Woe is me".

It is better to just get up if you neither *want* nor *need* to sleep; it is especially preferable to the often self-fulfilling pronouncement "I can't sleep". These three words are the *swiss army knife* of problem sleep: at once assessment, complaint, and prognosis. Unfortunately, this phrase performs none of these tasks especially well. Avoid it and your returning to sleep or getting up will be a more beneficial experience.

My son will sometimes complain that he can't sleep, even while lying there with his eyes wide open. And, as parents have from time immemorial, I tell him, as softly and soothingly as possible, "close your eyes and try". It is amazing sometimes how quickly sleep follows.

Let this advice for children serve as a model for you. Make sure you *try*. While the sandman may be a pleasant story to leave the waking world with, remember that it is a decidedly less romantic effort that actually encourages sleep to happen.

■　⬛　■

Ulterior motives

I see. I understand completely. This is about more than just regular schedules, following doctor's orders, and all that. You have ulterior motives for wanting to sleep. It's not just about rejuvenating your body and your senses. It goes beyond recharging your batteries.

You want to look better. Younger. You want to be happier and smarter. Have more energy. Be better at reasoning and problem solving. You want a leg up on the competition. You want to be the early bird that gets the worm for a change. And, at the risk of sounding like a snake oil salesman, I say to you, you can have all these things. And more. For the problem sleeper (and particularly those of the longtime variety) the benefits of a good night's sleep can almost be beyond imagining.

Personally, my family never took sleep seriously. It was a doctor that finally impressed on me that the body's requirements for sleep were just that: *requirements*. Sleep was necessary to be healthy, both mentally and physically. Granted, her approach was from the negative angle: what would happen to me if I *didn't* start to get enough sleep; but the message was effective nonetheless. Your own physician may not yet be so... well, enlightened. Or they may lack the background necessary to deal with your sleeplessness. It is up to you, then, to take the responsibility. Is there anything more important, really, than your health?

If your motives for overcoming your sleeplessness are more subtle, even selfish, that's perfectly okay; the more motives, the more motivated you will be to find a solution to your sleeplessness. In a similar scenario, consider that even when you are forced to go on a diet for all those important reasons (like cholesterol levels and blood pressure, and yes, even doctor's orders), somewhere in the background is a bathing suit with an improved you in

184

it, looking good. Whatever your motivation, the health and appearance benefits to be had by correcting your sleepless-ness (like those for improving your diet), are numerous and varied enough to make worthwhile your every ef-fort.

Go ahead, want more out of life. Feel more. Think more. Earn more. Accomplish more. Be more. Whatever your motivation is for seeking such things, you can't achieve them without sufficient sleep.

> *But suddenly he was freed from all pain, and felt fresh and healthy as if he had awakened from sleep, and when he opened his eyes he saw the maiden standing by him, snow-white, and fair as day.*
>
> *"Rise," said she, "and swing thy sword three times over the stairs, and then all will be delivered." And when he had done that, the whole castle was released from enchantment, and the maiden was a rich King's daughter.*
>
> The Brothers Grimm
> *The King's Son Who Feared Nothing*, 1812.

Upset

> *That we are not much sicker*
> *and much madder than we are*
> *is due exclusively to that most blessed*
> *and blessing of all natural graces,*
> *sleep.*
> Aldous Huxley

It has been said numerous times, in various ways, throughout this book, but it bears repeating here: just as an unsettled sleep cannot promote a peaceful mind, an unsettled mind cannot manage a peaceful sleep. Sleep is your reprieve, your respite from a waking existence that makes ever increasing demands on your mind and body. Make certain you provide sleep an environment in which it can flourish: not just a comfortable, secure physical surrounding, but a calm and serene mental state which makes genuinely welcome its arrival.

Vacation

One of the most adventurous things left
is to go to bed, for no one
lay a hand on our dreams.
E.V. Lucas

Your sleep is a chance to go on holiday every night. In your dreams you can escape from your mundane, daily worries, travel to new lands, meet new people; it needn't matter a bit that they actually exist or not. Not a vivid dreamer? That's okay; you rest, relax, and erase the cares of the day.

With such benefits imminent, you might try looking forward to bedtime each evening as you would a visit to a spa. Your nighttime **rituals**, the donning (or *doffing*, as the case may be) of your sleep attire, signals your embarking on an adventure. Far from an obligation or task forced upon you, you should look upon your evening slumber as an opportunity to ease the cares of your life. You can shut down, turn off, free yourself of worry, anxiety, tension, stress, and the multitude of other problems that can mark our waking existence.

Whatever the duration, this time is a gift; a gift of rest and relaxation given you each day. *Don't fail to take advantage of it!* Sleep the dreamless sleep, if you must, or the oft-interrupted variety, if that's all you're allowed to manage, but sleep. And remember that, even at it's worst, it is still sleep, and how bad can that be?

186

And if you find yourself actually *on* vacation, and having trouble sleeping?

A quite common scenario, given the changes in beds, **diet**, and schedule that vacations invariably bring with them. As we've discussed in **jet lag**, you may even find yourself in a different locale on a completely different day.

First and foremost is to be aware of your personal requirements regarding a regular sleep environment; (chances are, you've come to some conclusions already). How well do you take to changes in your sleep setting, or routine?

While making it "just like home" is probably an impossibility (and would you really want things to be just like home, anyway?), knowing what factors have the most influence on your sleep is more than half the battle. Can't eat too late in the evening and still sleep well? Need an opened window during the night, or an especially **firm** bed? Expect that such **rules** will still hold true, despite your unusual location, and take the steps (as much as possible) to provide them.

But expect that there will be plenty of changes, too, beyond your **control**. Besides the time change, be aware that you will probably eat more, and different foods than you may be accustomed to, and generally later in the day. You'll drink more, especially more alcoholic or caffeinated beverages, which can also affect your sleep. And the type and quality of the bed and **pillows** you will be sleeping on may be less than ideal.

Driving trips can mean that peculiar fatigue borne of inactivity; that phenomena of being *dead tired, with energy to burn* can be a real sleep wrecker. If you're planning on spending extended hours behind the wheel, try to incorporate regular stops that involve some kind of physical activity, if only to keep things circulating. After reaching your destination, you may be on your feet more, since **walking** is one of the best ways to appreciate a different place; this can increase your need for sleep. Your overall level of activity (physical and mental) will probably be higher, since you may be trying to accomplish as much as possible during your stay. And don't be surprised if, even if you're unaccustomed to it, an occasional **nap** is in order.

> "...lie down to sleep a little on the green grass after the fashion of knights-errant, so as to be fresher when day comes and the moment arrives for attempting this extraordinary adventure you are looking forward to..."

Or not. Vacations can be the ultimate excuse to experience life differently; there may literally be no limit of things to see, smell, taste, and appreciate. In such cases the last thing you may want to do is spend an hour or two in your hotel room, napping. There are those other vacations, of course, designed purely for the pursuit of leisure and relaxation, in such situations you may well be sleeping on the beach, by the pool, or logging a couple of hours back in the room in preparation for extended after-hours revelries.

In either case, knowing your body's needs and your established sleep habits and preferences can go a long way to insuring you get the sleep you need while on vacation. At the very least, you can avoid those behaviors contradictory to your established **sleep hygiene**; after all, while everything else may be completely different, (and *Vive la difference*, as they say in France), *you* are still *you*.

> "What art thou talking about dismounting or sleeping for?" said Don Quixote... "Sleep thou who art born to sleep, or do as thou wilt, for I will act as I think most consistent with my character."
>
> Miguel de Cervantes
> *Don Quixote*, 1615.

188

Valentine

*Care and sorrow and sleepless nights
are the lot of lovers.*
Washington Irving
Alhambra, 1832.

It happened. Caught off guard, with your defenses down (or even with them *up*, for that matter), you've been struck by Cupid's arrow. You're not thinking straight. You can't eat. You can't sleep. You're sick... with desire. Why, *you're in love*.

Congratulations on being willing to give so of yourself, to make yourself vulnerable. Be happy that you've found someone worthy of your attention (even if they prove later to be otherwise).

Hopefully your love is reciprocated: unrequited love is a notorious sleep stealer. But since not being absolutely certain of another's feelings is often (quite inextricably) tied to love, anyone's sleep can be in danger of suffering from such uncertainty. For the sake of your sleep (and your budding romance, for that matter), don't dwell on the uncertainties, especially to the point where it interferes with either your rest *or* your relationship.

Even if your love gives every indication of being one of the world's greatest, don't allow its prospects to distract you from your slumber: you'll need your strength to deal with this condition, among the most wonderful (and challenging) life has to offer. Unfortunately, time spent in reverie does not count as sleep. I *would* say to set a time limit to think about your beloved before retiring each night, but what is time to someone in love?

Others far more able than I have attempted, with varying success, to tackle the intricacies of love in print. Even within this narrow focus of sleep I will only offer the following recommendations: that being aware of the various factors that could influence your sleep must undoubtedly include those of love; to remember that late nights will certainly have an effect on your waking hours; that the often stimulative effects of a new love are no substitute for sleep; and that any thrashing around in the sheets should be *with* the object of your desire, not *over* them. And, finally, that if your relationship *does* have the misfortune to end, it will be not a moment too soon and will ultimately be for the best.

> *I had fallen violently in love with a girl... I fell into a regular fever, could think of nothing else; ...and my own conscience despising me for my uncontrollable weakness, made me so nervous and sleepless that I really thought I should become insane.*
>
> William James
> *The Varieties of Religious Experience*, 1902.

Vary

Do something different. *Anything*. It's okay; you don't have to ask anyone's permission. Especially after several sleepless nights.

While there are those sleep experts who feel consistency is the one immutable requirement of a sleep program, I can't help but think of all those casino gamblers gone bust, victims of that mind set that has them willingly repeating failure in pursuit of success, and all because their luck *just has to change*.

It doesn't, of course; and is there any good reason why your sleep troubles should be held up for nightly repetition or emulation, while deep, satisfying sleep remains elusive? If things are going well (and particularly if your sleep **ritual** has you relaxed and prepared for imminent slumber), then by all means, *stick with it*.

But at the same time, if exceedingly long periods awaiting sleep, numerous or regular awakenings during the night, or unsatisfying sleep **quality** continues to plague you, *do something about it.*

Make a change. Any change. You probably have, at this point, developed enough awareness of your sleep patterns and requirements to significantly and positively affect your situation. Even if you haven't (yet), your efforts to improve your sleep by changing things around a bit may unwittingly correct some situation contributing to your sleeplessness. Additionally, an occasional emphasis on variety can help avoid the performance anxiety that has a way of developing after several nights of unsatisfying sleep. And finally, if the situation warrants it, efforts at variety can help make clear the need for the help of a medical professional, even a sleep specialist.

At the very least, making changes means you are taking an active part in seeking better sleep; and that step, though basic, is nonetheless necessary to ending your sleeplessness. Good luck.

> *...it is safer to change many things, than one. Examine thy customs of diet, sleep, exercise, apparel, and the like; and try, in any thing thou shalt judge hurtful, to discontinue it, by little and little...*
>
> Francis Bacon
> *Essays*, 1601.

Versatility

Pursuing variety in your sleep options is, of course, only half of the equation; *you* are the other half. The human half. If you have only recently made inroads into your sleeplessness, you may be fearful that changes will upset the program, and jeopardize the progress you have made.

Don't be. As you become a better sleeper, have confidence that you are more adaptable to alternate sleep environments. Don't misunderstand: you may never reach that point where you can sleep well on a red-eye cross-country flight, or not awaken repeatedly during the night while tent camping; but you should take comfort in the fact that few of us ever do.

The mind is its own place, and in itself
Can make a heav'n of hell, a hell of heav'n.
John Milton
Paradise Lost, 1667.

While everything may be easier when things happen as expected, life is not especially based on consistency. Recognize that your sleep patterns and habits are just that, and the elements that make them up are not necessarily *requirements* for you to sleep.

As we have noted, consistency can be a double-edged sword; what feels comfortable can eventually become customary, what is familiar becomes the expected. Exceptions to this routine can be a source of anxiety, in sleep and in life. Rather than risk the discomfort and uncertainty that change can mean, you might want to view your versatility, your ability to handle change with aplomb, as a quality to be developed.

Become adept at adapting. Ultimately it is easier to learn to tack with the changing winds, and bob on the surface of the growing waves, than to expect smooth seas at all times. By becoming more easygoing, you leave yourself far less vulnerable to the anxieties that accompany our daily lives.

Any change, from a transit strike to a new desk assignment to the closing of your favorite restaurant, can produce discomfort, unhappiness, and even anxiety; but it's up to you to not lose any sleep over it.

I see nothing, not so much as in a dream, in a
wish, wheron I could set up my rest; variety only,
and the possession of diversity, can satisfy me;
that is, if anything can.
Montaigne
Essays, 1580-88.

192

Waiting up

She had no inclination to sleep; she was waiting, and such waiting was wakeful. But she closed her eyes; she believed that as the night wore on she should hear a knock at her door...

Henry James
Portrait of a Lady, 1881.

It's a hard thing to suffer through. Your mate had to work late at the office. Your teenager is out on a first date, or out with friends to a party. Whatever the reason or function, they said they'd be home at a certain time. And they're not. So you're left to wait up.

There are good reasons for wanting to be awake when they finally arrive home. But recognize that it's not necessarily a black mark on your parenting skills or comment on your relationship if you choose to sleep, either. You *do* have a choice.

I stress this because the one thing you should not do is lie there in bed, eyes closed but listening: to every car on the road, door opening or closing, every siren in the distance. Wait up or sleep. That's all there is to it. Your worrying will not get them home any faster or safer.

There are advantages to being awake when they finally get home; if only to note the actual time and their condition when they arrive. In such cases, sleeping in a location where they must necessarily awaken you can allow you to sleep *and* greet their arrival.

But save any recriminations and lecturing, even if needed, until **morning**; that is the time to decide the best course of action. Waiting up can leave you too fatigued, stressed, and emotional to properly deal with the situation; you may end up saying, and doing, something you later regret. And the last thing you want to do is apologize to the person that just kept you waiting up all night!

Walking
(and other sleep activities)

*Since his Majesty went into the field, I have
seen her rise from her bed, throw her
nightgown upon her, unlock her closet, take
forth paper, fold it, write upon't, read it,
afterwards seal it, and again return to bed;
yet all this while in a most fast sleep.*

William Shakespeare
Macbeth, 1606.

Although this book is more about attaining sleep
than sleep disorders, ambulatory sleep disturbances are
common enough to make them worthy of mention here.
Though fewer than 1 in 5 persons is ever affected, and
most exhibiting the tendency outgrow it by their teens, as
an object of portrayal in our popular culture sleepwalking has attained a remarkable level of awareness.

Sleepwalking (*somnambulism*) is an arousal disorder type of *parasomnia*, sleep intrusive disorders charac-
terized by disruptive sleep-related events. It is more common in children than in adults, and boys more than girls.
It tends to run in families, and while other medical and
psychiatric disorders, as well as other sleep disorders, may
be present, they do not seem to be connected to the symptom. Episodes can range in severity from an occasional
sitting up in bed to regular, even nightly, ramblings about
the house and grounds; some sleepwalkers are prone to
going outside, to the point of even attempting to drive a
car!

In children (and to a lesser extent, adults), the behavior is most often associated with fatigue, prior sleep
problems, and anxiety or stress. Techniques that have
proven successful in reducing the incidence and severity
of the condition include: avoiding getting overtired, self-
hypnosis, and relaxation and other stress reduction exercises. Since sleepwalking in adults, and particularly *adult*

onset cases, can often be associated with brain or personality disorders, seizures, and medication reactions, trained medical personnel *should* be consulted for anything other than the isolated episode.

The characteristic blank look of the sleepwalker, as well as their usual amnesia regarding the proceedings, has made it the stuff of imagination. Misconceptions abound: the agitation, confusion, and even terror often demonstrated by the awakened sleepwalker has no doubt contributed to the erroneous assumption that you should never rouse a sleepwalker; while the idea (perhaps mere rationalization) that sleepwalkers never injure themselves while sleepwalking is similarly false.

In fact, one would do well to use common sense as a guide to living with a sleepwalker. Doors and windows should be kept closed and locked to avoid wandering, floors kept clear of items that could cause tripping, and the sleepwalker's bedroom should be kept on the ground floor, to avoid a possibly unpleasant stair situation.

As to a cure, thankfully, most never need to think in those terms: their episodes are mild or infrequent enough, if they don't outgrow them entirely. However, if sleepwalking episodes are regular, behaviors highly unusual and injuries (or the threat of them) common, *don't delay*; see a sleep specialist forthwith.

Because the danger is real: people *can* and *do*, get hurt while sleepwalking. And not always just the people doing the walking: a man recently went on trial for repeatedly stabbing his wife and then drowning her. His (unsuccessful) defense? He was "sleepwalking" at the time.

Parasomnia research has identified a related behavior, and given it a name that both describes and classifies it: *nocturnal eating syndrome*. Those suffering from this condition get out of bed in the middle of the night to eat. What makes it different than the usual midnight snack, besides that trancelike state characteristic of ambulatory sleep disorders, is that the person often consumes startlingly large amounts and unusual combinations of food. Not surprisingly, the person has no memory of the incident. The lasting effects of this syndrome seem to be minor: a disruption of the sleep cycle (though can this be considered minor, really?), and a similar disruption of the daytime eating cycle. And, not surprisingly, a significant, though previously inexplicable, weight gain.

Which points us to an altogether different relationship between sleep and walking. As we discussed in **diet**, (and will analyze further in just a few pages) a body that works better tends to sleep better. Walking is an excellent way to get your body to function the way it's supposed to, particularly if you don't have (or have been avoiding) a regular exercise routine.

Since the amount of calories that walking can burn rivals those of more strenuous activities, weight loss, as well as improved respiration, circulation, and overall physical condition, can all result from a regular walk.

But our goal here is not aerobic conditioning as much as a regular, stress relieving, yet still physical, activity. A walk can be a good way to relax after a stressful day, help digest your evening meal, and generally recondition your body to its natural processes, which, once the sun is down, is increasingly gearing toward sleep.

And if you do have a tendency to walk *while sleeping*, an evening walk while awake can be invaluable in preventing it from occurring later.

> I think it will be best for her to go to bed tired out physically, so I shall take her for a long walk by the cliffs to Robin Hood's Bay and back. She ought not to have much inclination for sleep-walking then.
>
> Bram Stoker
> *Dracula*, 1897.

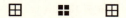

Want

*'Now look here, you- you thick-headed beast,'
replied the Rat, really angry, 'this must stop.
Not another word, but scrape- scrape and
scratch and dig and hunt round...if you want
to sleep dry and warm to-night, for it's our
last chance!'*

Kenneth Grahame
The Wind in the Willows, 1908.

Think of it as the antecedent of **try**. It's not enough
to stretch, yawn, and announce to the room at large, "I
think I'll call it a night"; you have to really *want* to go to
sleep. It won't do to be lying in bed, thinking you "should"
be asleep: if you don't want to, no amount of exercises,
techniques, games, or **herbs** will put you there.

If you're in the middle of having fun, but see that
it's getting late, remember that you are no longer a child,
constrained by a designated bedtime; that's one of the
bona fide perks of adulthood. By all means, stay up until
you are ready for bed. If you must be up early, use that
adult sense of **responsibility** you have developed to gauge
just how late you can (or *should*, anyway) stay up. It's
your call; you are the one having to get up and function
the next day.

If it's something *keeping* you up, despite your body's
readiness, determine if it's anything that can be postponed:
television programming that can be taped, paperwork that
can be done tomorrow, a book that can be continued
while in bed. Sometimes not wanting to go to bed changes
once the inducement for staying awake is removed.

In my own case, it was a little more complex. A job
transfer had me starting work earlier, and getting home
later. Wanting to make up for the time I was apart from
my family, I got into the habit of staying up later than I
should have. I wasn't ready to end my day: my play time

with the family was still going on! And, with the help(?) of caffeinated drinks and other measures, I would manage to stay awake. Unfortunately, the ramifications of this behavior, especially the long term ones, were soon made apparent.

The solution was an unexpected one— I started going to the gym after work. Granted, this was an extra hour or so, 3 or 4 times a week, away from my family. But instead of arriving home exhausted, marginally functioning and in need of caffeine, I was getting my second wind. I had more energy and stamina, and rather than dragging around, I was playing and roughhousing with my young son. Our time together was more productive, and we both went to bed at a more reasonable hour. And once there, I was able to fall asleep more easily, without the need to overcome the effects of stimulants.

I remember all those times I had lain in bed, thinking I should be out there, interacting with my family. At such times, I couldn't sleep, no matter how tired I was. When I eventually managed to get what I felt was lacking, I had no trouble falling asleep: not until I was able to really *want* sleep could I manage it.

Wanting to sleep is not just an indicator of your general attitude toward sleep, it can be a predictor of your success in attaining it. Don't go to bed solely because you feel you *should*; far too many times it serves only to highlight the difference between going to *bed* and going to *sleep*.

*If you choose to sleep, I wish you goodnight;
but if you prefer talking, I recommend you
to talk of fighting or of fair ladies.*
Thomas Bulfinch
Romance of the Middle Ages, 1863.

Weather

Heavy with the heat and silence
Grew the afternoon of Summer;
With a drowsy sound the forest
Whispered round the sultry wigwam...

And the guests of Hiawatha,
Weary with the heat of Summer,
Slumbered in the sultry wigwam....
Henry Wadsworth Longfellow
The Song of Hiawatha, 1855.

It is so hot and humid that you can only hope you make it to the end of this hellish day, when you can throw your weary body down in a heap and sleep. But once in bed, sleep proves elusive: you manage only to toss and turn in sweating wakefulness.

While it may be true that people talk about the weather only because they're unable to do anything about it, when your sleep is at stake, sometimes you have to take a much more *proactive* approach. If you can manage it, an air conditioner (at least a bedroom window model) is worth the effort and expense; if you can't, take any steps necessary to attain the comfort you need to sleep. If sprinkling the sheets with water, electric fans, and exposing as much bared skin as possible are all you can manage, then do it! A cloud of cornstarch can help with the stickiness. A cool or cold shower, right before bed, can provide enough temporary relief to allow you to fall asleep; a similar bath can give benefits that last slightly longer.

Of course, that other season can mean sleep discomfort as well, though it is far easier to drag another blanket onto the bed than cool a sweltering body. The nightcap (the one that goes on your head, not the rum toddy) has been with us for hundreds of years as a way to help keep your head warm in cold weather, but recent research indicates that additional bedwear may be even more effective at maintaining proper sleep temperature. Socks, and gloves or mittens, helped laboratory subjects both fall asleep faster and awaken less often during the night, presumably by minimizing the temperature variations that occur as part of the sleep cycle. Of course, such *accoutrements* can interfere with my preferred method of maintaining the proper warmth for slumber: snuggling. But then, any port in a storm...

The important thing to keep in mind here is to not be caught unaware regarding the weather's changes and the ways it can affect your optimal sleep environment. In this regard, it is equally important, if not *more* important, to monitor the usually temperate seasons of Spring and Fall for weather and temperature changes that can compromise your sleep. An icicle dangling off your nose may be a sure sign to pull up the down comforter, but a night where the mercury drops 30 or more degrees between retiring and waking can be tougher to deal with.

As has been discussed, even small, seemingly inconsequential nighttime concerns can mean disturbed, and thereby unsatisfying, sleep. Merely being aware of changes in the weather, and the possibility they will affect your sleep, can be enough to prevent their compromising your comfort. And your **comfort**, as you have learned, is foremost when it comes to sleep.

> *They could get bedding at a secondhand store, she explained; and they would not need any, while the weather was so hot- doubtless they would all sleep on the sidewalk such nights as this, as did nearly all of her guests.*
> Upton Sinclair
> *The Jungle*, 1906.

Work

It's all in a day's work.
Anonymous,
c. 18th century.

Or is it? In this day and age, especially given the rapid advances in technology, the end of a day's work has become increasingly indistinct. Although the average length of the work week has changed little since the mid 1970's, the number of workers putting in a very long work-week (exceding the standard 40 hours by a full 8 hour day or more) has increased significantly; and such a schedule has become almost expected in many occupations. In addition, e-mail, cell phones, pagers, and other personal electronics have made it more difficult to avoid the employer, customer, or other work-related associate making demands of you *outside* the workplace.

When you add to the mix telecommuters, those working for others out of their home, or working for themselves in a home-based business, the possibilities for work intruding on personal time, and especially those hours intended for sleep, has increased exponentially.

Contrary to appearances, that time in the quiet of late evening is *not* ideal for finishing up a project, nor is it perfect for getting a head start on work you know awaits you in the morning.

Sleep after toil,
port after stormy seas,
Ease after war,
death after life
does greatly please.
Edmund Spenser
The Faerie Queene, 1590.

As we have noted earlier, if you must bring your work home with you, set a specific time *with a fixed end-*

point for working on it. Your goal should be to stop well before bedtime, to allow sufficient time for both winding down and your pre-sleep ritual. A less desirable second choice would be stopping *at* the actual hour for bed. If your sleep and overall health are important to you, though, you should consider it unacceptable (at least, on a regular basis) to let work intrude into that time dedicated for sleep.

Remember, too, that the end of work involves more than just putting the pencil down and standing up from your desk. Don't allow your thoughts and energies to drift to business matters just because you're lying, undisturbed, in bed: such cogitations *are* a disturbance, as far as your sleep is concerned, as much as any phone ringing or beeper going off.

> *My health and my good spirits flagged... Besides my daylight servitude, I served over again all night in my sleep, and would awake with terrors of imaginary false entries, errors in my accounts, and the like.*
>
> Charles Lamb
> *The Last Essays of Elia*, 1833.

The modern workplace can present additional problems, particularly when it's in the worker's own home. If you're one of the growing number of people doing business from your home, a few precautions can help protect your precious sleep.

Most important is to keep your workplace out of the bedroom. If you don't, you could very well end up sleeping when you should be working, and working when you are supposed to be sleeping. If it's at all possible, write your bills, file your invoices, or crunch your numbers in some other area of your home. Not only is the temptation too great to "just do a little work" before bed (easily becoming *instead of* bed), often just *seeing* your work area can be enough to trigger the anxieties, con-

202

cerns, and the mental listing of tasks associated with any business; no good can come of *that* happening while you're preparing for bed.

Keeping business out of the bedroom can be especially critical if you are sleeping with your business partner (when they're also your *life* partner). Though that quiet time while lying in bed may seem your only chance to talk, it may be your only chance to do several other things, as well; one of which is sleep. Don't neglect the need for discussion (it's one of the things that successful businesses encourage) just make sure you set aside the time for it during the course of the day.

If you have your own business, make a foremost concern your *quality of life,* both for you and your family. Most people running their own business do so, in some measure, for the independence it promotes; demonstrate your own independence by putting an enjoyable, satisfying life (one that includes satisfying *sleep)* near the top of the expected profits. Besides, you won't be able to effectively manage those business meetings and deals without your requisite sleep.

No matter where you toil, work hard at work; it is one of the ingredients of success. But recognize that the more *satisfying* your work experience is, the less chance it will interfere with your sleep (and vice versa). Because at bedtime, you have no business thinking about business.

> *...when the day's work is done, we go on thinking of losses and gains, we plan for the morrow, we even carry our business cares to bed with us, and toss and worry over them when we ought to be restoring our racked bodies and brains with sleep. We burn up our energies with these excitements, and either die early or drop into a lean and mean old age...*
> Mark Twain
> *The Innocents Abroad,* 1869.

Workout

Although it's got the word in its name, it needn't be. Work, that is. Sure, summoning the right attitude, preparing your equipment bag, fighting traffic, and finding parking can be a tremendous effort, and all that before you've even set foot in the gym!

But that's one kind of workout. And since *any* kind of exercise will help you to sleep better (a big claim, I know), anyone can develop a beneficial exercise program suited to their particular needs and abilities.

It needn't even *be* a program. Particularly if you are someone who hasn't participated lately or regularly, an exercise regimen is best initiated through a series of small steps. The first? See your doctor, both to identify factors that could limit your level of activity and to establish a baseline to chart your progress.

Then, start with a *mental* stretch. Don't think of exercise as some onerous task, the physical equivalent of castor oil. It is best (and, surprisingly, *easiest*) when thought of as a general approach to life. If it's left to you to buy a club membership and a bunch of workout outfits, or worse, a roomful of home exercise equipment, in order to derive the benefits of fitness, you probably won't do it. And that's not intended as criticism, but an assessment of human nature. If you can, will, or already do these things, *great*.

If you don't, try this: the next time you have to visit another floor in your building, take the stairs rather than the elevator. Or go ahead and park your car on the outskirts of the lot, rather than make another pass to find a spot close to the door. Walk to the corner mailbox, instead of driving to the post office, to mail your letter. Walk with your child to school in the morning (if they're of an age that *allows* it): you might even learn something new about them!

The idea is, that by using your body a bit more for the concerns of daily life, you begin conditioning it for more organized, or directed, exercise. In order to be *active* you must first *act*, and while there are all kinds of excuses for not taking part in a formal exercise program, there are few, if any, for not leading a generally more active life. Any kind of physical movement will help your heart, your weight, your attitude, and yes, your sleep.

But once you've reached that point, you may be looking for more. Still dreading that gym/workout situation? Take a different tack. Play tennis? No? Good. Instructional classes are a great way to be introduced to a sport or physical activity: the emphasis on learning helps keep a ceiling on the exertion, especially at the start, and it gives you a viable substitute to the gym for the rest of your life.

Look to *alternatives* to traditional exercise: they can provide health benefits in ways that may better suit your personality. Dancing (particularly *ballroom* or *swing*, for instance) can help bring about good heath while expanding your social life. Yoga is a classic form of "exercise" that includes stretching and slow movement. The physical *and* mental benefits are tremendous, and you can, literally and figuratively, do it for life.

Another exercise that fits in the "alternative" category (at least in this country) is Tai-Chi, the ancient Far East martial arts discipline that goes beyond self defense: while the fluid, stylized movements promote strength and flexibility, the emotional state evinced is decidedly meditative. In China, young and old alike fill public squares and parks for sessions. And while I open myself up to charges of nepotism (my twin brother Joshua is a martial arts master and a director of the Boston Kung Fu/Tai-Chi Institute), research has found this among the most beneficial of exercises for seniors.

It really doesn't matter what form of exercise you choose, from riding your bike to work to taking a walk after dinner. *Start moving.* Whatever your limitations, strive to improve your physical capabilities; the benefits to your sleep will surely prove commensurate.

> *What with plenty to eat and fresh air and exercise that was taken as it pleased him, he would waken from his sleep and start off not knowing what to do with his energy, stretching his arms, laughing, singing old songs of home that came back to him.*
>
> Upton Sinclair
> *The Jungle*, 1906.

Woulda'
Coulda'
Shoulda'

> *God knows, I'm not the thing I should be, nor am I even the thing I could be.*
> Robert Burns
> *Posthumous Pieces*, 1799.

You could have been somebody. Done something. You could have, should have, made more of your life. You may have made a mistake; gotten mixed up with the wrong crowd, did things that weren't *you*. You may have let the love of your life get away, or screwed up that real opportunity to get ahead.

And now you're paying the price. Maybe not every night, but often enough that you're not sleeping any the better for it. As has been noted earlier, the dark of night has a way of giving strength to thoughts such as these, thoughts that, in the light of day, seem somehow diminished, of lesser importance.

Recognize the part that *perspective* plays in this scenario: though the essential facts may be correct, your interpretation may be colored by the *noir* setting; the conclusions you come to while lying in bed and those of morning may be different...well, as different as night and day.

Realize, too, that things often appear more straight-forward in recollection than they were in occurrence; the flat mental photograph of memory renders few details of the intricately woven, densely textured fabric that is our life.

And if it's not just perception? If these nighttime regrets are a sign that something is wrong, or missing? Do something about it. Either get up, out of bed, at that very moment (if a dramatic change in your life isn't worth missing one night's sleep, I don't know what is), or get some sleep immediately, in anticipation of **morning**. Then figure out what it is you need to correct, or are missing. Consider your goals, your dreams, and the best way to achieve them. Seek the help and advice of professionals, if you need to; when the way is so confusing, there is certainly no shame in finding a competent guide to help you determine the best route.

As we have mentioned earlier, don't offer your sleep-lessness up as some penance for what you did, or didn't do, in the past; if effecting a positive change is what you need in your life, this behavior is counterproductive, at best. Think in terms of solutions, not absolution.

Be aware that, often, seemingly small changes can yield impressive results, in your life and in your sleep. The number of techniques you can use to bring about a positive change are many. Just remember: regret *can* sometimes be a good thing; but only if it spurs you to positive change. If it's just keeping you from sleep, it's an emotion you can certainly do without.

> *"I could've been a contender, I could've had class*
> *and been somebody, Real class. Instead of a bum,*
> *let's face it, which is what I am..."*
> *Terry Malloy*
> *(played by* Marlon Brando)
> *On The Waterfront, 1954.*

Write

If your mistakes, your wishes, your dreams, or your frustrations are keeping you from sleeping, write them down. Having to come up with actual *words* to convey and communicate such ideas can help order your thoughts, and make concrete that which may exist in a less tangible, and thereby less manageable, form.

Don't worry that you're not witty or facile enough with words or language. This is for *you*, not the public; just the act of doing it means success. And don't agonize over spelling or grammar. Just get it down on paper.

How is this different from a **journal**? For one thing, you don't have to feel any *obligation* to write. It can be one thing that's troubling you, or one desire that has to be expressed; it doesn't have to be continued, or ongoing, or reflect your feelings three weeks hence. You needn't even keep the result: after you write it down, you may very well throw it away.

Say things on paper that you could never say in person. If you're creative, invent a thinly veiled character that says them for you, ala a *roman a clef*. Cover the page with words of protest, then toss it in the trash as the ultimate act of defiance. Or send it to the editor of your newspaper. By writing things down, you can let go of fears, defeats, and worries, and bring into focus concerns, aspirations, and desires.

It can be as simple as a list. As complex as a novel. Putting words down on paper is a tool readily available to *all* of us, regardless of our training or skill, background or social status. And among its many benefits can certainly be counted the **ability** to help us sleep.

The right to write badly
was the privilege we widely used.
Isaac Babel
Speech at First Writers Congress, 1934.

Writer's block

And if you already write, and find yourself (hopefully temporarily) unable to manage it? Don't overlook the relationship of sleep to words in this regard, either. Artistic creations too numerous to count have had their origins in the artist's dream state: many a creative logjam of the conscious mind has been freed by the flow of the subconscious mind in sleep. So, for possible material, attune your writer's ear to the voices of your dreams, as well as to the dialogue of the real world.

> *I explained the phenomena as partly due to explicitly conscious processes of thought and will, but as due largely also to the subconscious incubation and maturing of motives deposited by the experiences of life. When ripe, the results hatch out, or burst into flower.*
>
> William James
> *The Varieties of Religious Experience*, 1902.

X-Ray

> *And at night I close my eyes, and I can still see through my own eyelids! I'd give anything, anything, to have dark...*
>
> Dr. James Xavier
> (*played by* Ray Milland)
> *X; The Man with the X-Ray Eyes*, 1963.

Yes, of course. This entry *is* in response to the alphabetical format of this book. But, as one of the moments of true horror in a drive-in screamer that has the protagonist, for much of the film, looking through people's clothes, it establishes a definite benchmark, as well.

He can't sleep at night because he sees right through his eyelids! As sleep problems go, this must certainly rank among the very worst. So no matter how bad things get, take some comfort in the fact that you don't have Dr. X's problem.

And while you're at it, give some thanks to your eyelids; a more important (at least in terms of sleep), yet more *taken for granted* part of the body I can't imagine.

Yawn

> *[He] became aware that his lower jaw was uncontrollably forming a yawn. He pulled his whiskers to cover the yawn, and shook himself together. But soon after he became aware that he was dropping asleep and on the very point of snoring.*
>
> Leo Tolstoy
> *Anna Karenina*, 1873-76.

Forget what you may have heard about a yawn just being an automatic physical response to the body's need for oxygen. A yawn can have a psychological basis, as well, and can be triggered by impatience, frustration, or boredom. It can be used to show, intentionally or otherwise, disdain or unhappiness. A yawn can be used to mask (or attempt to, anyway) a lie.

And it can help you to sleep.

I know what you're thinking: "a yawn means you're sleepy. The work's already been done." But we're not looking here at yawn as *effect* as much as a possible *cause*; exploring the possibility that a yawn can, if not actually *make* you sleepy, at least help you to that mental state conducive to sleep.

Consider the effect of a boring lecture on a crowded classroom. While a lack of adequate ventilation may be contributing to the increasing number of yawns seen throughout the room (a common situation), it could also be a practical demonstration of "catching a yawn". This syndrome was considered the stuff of folk wisdom, until recent studies of baboon behavior bore it out: the "group

210

yawn" signals that they are settling down for the night. We may just yawn as an indication of the same, and others, like the baboons, yawn back as a sign they got the message.

> *So at last, with a sigh and a yawn, he gave it up. It seemed to him that the noon recess would never come... The drowsing murmur of the five and twenty studying scholars soothed the soul like the spell that is in the murmur of bees.*
>
> Mark Twain
> *Tom Sawyer*, 1876.

But let's take this connection one step further. If a yawn can indeed be a conditioned response, why not tap into those countless times (a lifetime's worth) you've yawned, and sleep soon followed?

Go ahead. Try it. But don't give it just a weak, half-hearted effort: yawn like it's really happening. This is no time to be polite: open your mouth wide, and stretch your arms skyward, your hands curled in gentle fists. Think about how genuinely tired you are, and how nice it would be to be lying in bed, asleep.

If you're like me, this *faux* yawn turns into a real one surprisingly often, and I doubt it's because I'm such a talented actress. I think the body is just naturally responding to the stimulus, irrespective of whether it was initiated consciously or unconsciously; like a clock striking the hour whether it corresponds to the time in Greenwich or not. Of course, it's up to you to keep the momentum toward sleep going past this point, but segueing into your pre-sleep ritual is a natural; another behavior that, genuine or otherwise, has the body thinking sleep. Sweet dreams.

> *"I don't see why God made any night; day is so much pleasanter," said Nan thoughtfully.*
> *"It's to sleep in," answered Rob, with a yawn.*
> *"Then do go to sleep," said Nan pettishly.*
>
> Louisa May Alcott
> *Little Men*, 1871.

211

Zero

Hast never come to thee an hour,
A sudden gleam divine, precipitating, bursting all these
bubbles, fashions, wealth?
These eager business aims- books, politics, art, amours,
To utter nothingness?
Walt Whitman
Leaves of Grass, 1855.

It seems an unlikely goal. Nothing. Nil. Zero. Zilch. But for many it is the Grail they seek, the answer to their foremost need, the solution to their sleeplessness.

Become a blank page in an empty book. Forget about peaceful thoughts, soothing thoughts, relaxing thoughts. The goal here is *no* thoughts: no worries, no fears, nothing. In this way there is nothing (relaxing or otherwise) to keep you awake, to demand your attention; nothing to call you back once you move nearer the edge of sleep.

Your body still exists, has emotions and feelings, but you are separated from it. You are floating weightless, detached and numb to its sensations. There is no more striving, no more wanting, no more denying. There is no more trying; not even to sleep. You are nothing. Zero.

You may as well sleep; there is nothing more to do in this world. With utter confidence that you will ultimately awaken, you step off, and begin a slow drift toward sleep. Nothing can stand in your way, because *you* are nothing, with no real ties to everything you are leaving behind. The only thing you have to lose is yourself, to that fathomless void of sleep.

[He] would rather...sleep forever in the trade-winds under the southern stars, wandering over the dark purple ocean, with its purple sense of solitude and void...it was the most unearthly he had felt.

Henry Adams
The Education of Henry Adams, 1907.

212

Zzzzz...

This shorthand for sleep is an altogether appropriate ending for this book. And by way of conclusion, I offer here some reminders, suggestions, and explanations (if you're not asleep already, that is...).

It has been my goal to make *user friendly* a branch of scientific study that can seem imposing, and, at times, even arbitrary and contradictory. Suffering sleeplessness can, in itself, mean increased stress, without adding the pressure that negotiating jargon-laden scientific treatises can sometimes bring. The alphabetical organization of the Sleep Book is a device to make accessible (and I hope, entertaining), just some of the tremendous amount of information available on the subject.

As your knowledge and interest grow, though, even (*especially?*) after your sleep shows improvement, you may want to explore other sources of information. Sleep research, at this point, is the stuff of promising developments as much as earthshaking discoveries, and while this is due in part to the still-formative stage of the research and its associated methodologies, much of it may prove attributable to the individual nature of sleep itself.

What does this mean for you? Primarily that you will want to stay up-to-date: like so many findings in the health sciences (particularly concerning diet and nutrition), information that is one day presented as definitive is often, soon after, thoroughly debunked. The more you know about sleep the more discerning you will be regarding future findings, recommendations, and their relevance to you.

The Internet is one good way to stay informed, reflective of the speed with which health information is being accumulated and disseminated. And despite the appearance of a shameless plug, (forget appearances, it *is* a shameless plug) The Sleep Book website (www.sleepbook.com, or www.howtosleep.com) is one way to help you stay current on research findings, link you to other sleep related sites, and provide a welcome place for you to rest your weary brain. While you're there, register for the newsletter; a convenient way to discover not just the latest developments, but what has worked for *others like you*. With this in mind, I welcome accounts from fellow travelers on the road to good sleep. You can write to the address on the copyright page of this book, or send an e-mail while visiting the website, and let me know how your journey goes.

And don't worry, if you're visiting the site in the middle of the night, about getting any lectures on what you *should* be doing at that hour...

If, even after our efforts here, your sleeplessness is persistent, long term, or recurring, I urge you again to *see a sleep specialist*. They can go far beyond what can be offered on the written page. Sometimes only a trained third party can identify conditions that would otherwise go undetected by the sleeper.

Just as your sleeplessness probably did not develop overnight, so may your response to it take some time and effort. For many, behavior modification is an ongoing process that can take a while merely to show results, let alone realize full benefits. For others, a quick trip to the family physician can resolve their apnea or their bedmate's snoring. You may find that developing a comprehensive program of physical and mental exercises, or finally resolving those unanswered personal needs or desires, provides the key to unlocking your sleeplessness.

Appreciate the process as much as the result. Realize that there is as much, and more, to learn about yourself as about your sleeplessness, and that the two are inextricably wedded. As we said at the very start, think of your efforts to overcome your problem sleep as a journey; and this book as an inspiring and informative guide book for your trip: what you will need to take with you, some of the must-sees along the way, and a thorough, if far from comprehensive, picture of where you should eventually end up.

Good luck on your journey, and sweet dreams always.

> *'I must say I don't understand your technicalities,'* she said; *'but I do your conclusion, and I don't like it... So I shall expect, after breakfast, to receive my first lesson. And then you shall lie down and sleep.'*
> Jack London
> *Sea Wolf*, 1904.

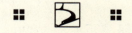

Index

A

accupressure 64
active sleepers 49
adaptability 191–192
addiction 119
adulthood 159
air purifier 72
airborne toxins 59
alarm clocks 20–21, 22,
    151, 158
alcohol 43, 82, 84, 131, 166,
    169, 187
allergens 70
allergies 24, 55, 71
ambulatory sleep distur-
    bances 194–196
analgesics 64
Andy Warhol's Sleep 111
anger 58, 79–80
animal dander 71
antacids 34
anti-allergens 127, 148
antihistamines 169
anxiety 9, 32, 43, 44, 79,
    186, 191, 192, 194, 202
apnea 19, 70, 149, 168
aroma therapy 55
aspirin 65
aural intrusions 153
autodidactism 143

B

baboons 211
basil 67
bath 42
bed(s) 23, 24, 49, 54, 108,

146, 187
bedclothes 72
bedroom 24, 30, 69, 71
bedtime 148
behavior modification 74,
    160, 214
belladonna 55
benzoin 67
bergamot 67
blindfold 40
body temperature 39, 115
booklights 156
books on tape 155
brain disorders 195
brain wave patterns 102
breathing 10, 147, 161
bruxism 12, 19, 149
buckwheat hull pillows
    139–140

C

cabin fever 99
caffeine 28, 65, 81-
    82, 166, 187, 198
calamint 67
California poppy 67
camphor 67
cannabis 67
carpet 71
catnip 67
cause(s) 8–9, 18, 94
chamomile 55, 66
change(s) 95, 192, 207
chanting 103

childhood 32, 159
childhood conditioning 92
children 49, 126, 183
chocolate 82
chronophobia 20, 159
circadian rhythm
    83, 84, 97, 115
circulation 139, 196
circulatory system 65
clinical depression 130
clock 20–21, 28, 149, 158–
    159
coffee 81, 86, 123,
    163, 177
color 29–31
comfort 23, 30, 133
compromise 126
computer 47, 173–174
conditioned response
    119, 211
consciousness 102, 171
control 25-26, 171
coping 27
counting 124–125
Crawford, Joan 182
crying 26, 61
Cupid 189
cure 27
curtained bed 16

D

danger 164–165
darkness 40, 104
datura 55
dawn simulating alarm
    clock 98
daydreaming 38
death 175
decision(s) 28, 54
decor 29

deep sleep 31–32
dehydration 19, 42, 65
delayed onset sleep 9, 70
dentist 13
dependence 119
depressant 42
diary 85
diet 33, 72, 120, 196
digestion 33
diurnal 115
down feather pillow 139
dreams 37-39, 55, 80, 121,
    186, 210
drugs, see narcotics
dust 71
dust mites 71

E

e-mail 173
ear aches 13
early risers 9
early bird 126
earplugs 153
efficiency 46, 107
electricity 99
eleven o'clock news 161
emotion 193
energy 198
entertainment 41
environment 23, 29, 30–
    32, 69, 70, 72, 104,
    152, 153, 187, 191, 200
espresso 82, 86
essential oil(s) 66, 127
eucalyptus 67
exercise 86, 169, 204–206
eye drops 48, 123
eyes 47

F

familial advanced sleep-
    phase syndrome 92
families 194
family bed 49-51
fatigue 194
fidgeting 52
firmness 53
florae 66
flowers 55
formaldehyde 71
frustration 7, 8, 25, 26 ,38,
    57, 131, 137, 138, 143
futon 54

G

garden 59–60
genetics 92
ginseng 67
glare 47
glaucoma 47
Goldilocks 23, 54
government 57–58
grinding your teeth 12–
    14, 172
    see also: bruxism
guilt 61, 172
Gumby 24

H

habits 86, 120, 129, 157
    188, 192
habituation 119
hammocks 63
headache(s) 13, 64, 65, 172
heartburn 19, 33
helichrysum italicum 55
herbs 28, 60, 65, 66, 84,
    119 127

heredity 92
hiatal hernia 33
honey 66
hops 67
Houdini, Harry 10
human growth hormone
    128
hunger 34
hygiene 69
hypnosis
    self hypnosis 10
hypoallergenic 70

I

ideal(s) 73, 130, 151, 162
imagination 74
impatience 137–138
infant(s) 100, 118
inhalation 66
inhalers 67
insomnia 145
inspiration 44
Internet 173–174, 213,214
interruptions 70, 76, 153
isometrics 84

J

jaw(s) 13
jet lag 83–85, 99
journal 78, 85, 109, 128,
    148

K

keepsake 89, 154
kimono 90
kindness 91
knack 91

218

L

lavender 55, 66, 67
leg cramps 19
lemon-balm 67
light 97–98, 104, 152
lists 141
location 157
love 189–190
lullabies 100

M

mantra 32, 102, 147
martial arts 205
masks 40, 104, 151
masseter muscles 13
mattress 23, 53- 54, 69, 148
medications 27, 65, 67,
    72, 165, 195
meditation 10, 59, 146, 205
melatonin 85
memories 89, 105
mental images 161
mildews 71
milk 28, 33
minerals 82
mineral deficiency 19
missing time 173–174
molds 71
Monroe, Marilyn 133
morning 109, 123, 148
motivation 185
movies 110–112
mud 112
muscle relaxants 13, 169
music 100, 113, 161

N

naps 49, 95
nap room 116
narcotics 118–120
natural 59
neroli 67, 127
neurological disorders 130
nicotine 65, 82
night guard 13, 172
nightcap 199
nightmares 120–122, 152
night owls 49, 126
nightshade 55
nightshirt 134
nocturnal eating syndrome
    195–196
nocturnal myoclonus 19
nutritional deficiencies 130

O

obstructive sleep apnea 168
oversleep 128
overweight 35

P

pain 65, 131-132
pain killers 131
pajamas 133-134
paperwork 197
parasomnia 194–196
passion 57, 58, 135
passionflower 67
patience 8, 28, 137–
    138, 162
patterns 151, 192
penance 172
personality disorders 195
petitgrain 67

pharmaceuticals 67
physical activity 196
physician 169
pillow(s) 23–24, 139–
140, 148, 172, 187
plans 141
plants 59–60, 66
politics 57–58
pollen 72
pollutants 59
popliteal region 97
post-work nap 117
pre-sleep 13, 15, 32, 85,
113, 138, 161, 162, 202
preferences 188
preparations 98
prescriptions 118, 181
primrose 67
programs 26, 142, 152, 163
progressive relaxation
61, 146–147, 161

Q

quality 7, 148–149, 152
quiet 21, 152–153
quilts 154

R

reading 155–156, 161
reason(s) 18, 123
regret 36, 79, 206-207
relax(ation) 11, 12, 17, 30,
59, 96, 108, 120, 146-
147, 153, 186, 194
religion 102
repetition 102
respiration 196
restless 52

ritual(s) 15, 32, 41, 85,
103, 113, 160-161, 162,
186, 190, 203, 211
rose(s) 55, 66, 67
routine 163, 187
rules 159, 162–163

S

safety 164
sandalwood 67
schedules 87, 117, 126, 187
201
security 89, 134, 160
seizures 195
self-hypnosis 10, 13, 194
serotonin 33
sex 135
shaking legs syndrome 149
shaking limbs 149
sheets 24
shift work 99
siestas 116
skullcap 67
sleep hygiene 129, 166–167
169
sleeping pills 118-120, 131,
169
sleepwalking 194–196
sneezing 71
snoring 19, 70, 157, 167,
172
sodas 81
somnambulism 194–196
spikenard 67
stimulant(s) 42, 198
stress 8, 13, 19, 64, 92,
120, 121, 122, 141, 186,
193, 194
reduction 120
reduction exercises 194

suggestibility 14
support 63, 112
surrender 25, see also:
    succumb 171
surroundings 29–
    31, 32, 70, 89, 186
sweet marjoram 67
symptoms 131

T

tai-chi 206
talking in sleep 19
tea 42, 81, 82
technology 202
television 41, 197
temperature 23, 90, 98, 200
temporomandibular joint
    disorders 13
tension 186
tinnitus 42
tragedy 26, 180–181
tranquilizers 127, 169
travel 117
tryptophan 33

U

ulterior motives 184–185

V

vacation 151, 186–188
valerian 67
ventilation 63, 69, 71
versatility 192
vetiver 67
visualization 74
vitamins 19, 82

W

waiting up 126, 193
walking 204
water 96
waterbeds 54
weather 199
wine 86
winter induced depression
    99
work 15, 201
work out 120, 204–206
  see also: exercise
world music 114
worry 186
write 62, 208

X

X-ray 209

Y

yawn 210
ylang-ylang oil 67
yoga 205

Acknowledgments

I would like to gratefully acknowledge the many writers, scientists, and philosophers whose reflections on the subject of sleep have contributed so much to this book. While every effort has been made to determine whether previously published material included herein required permission to quote, I make no claims of infallibility; I apologize for any oversights, and assure you that any necessary corrections will be made in future editions.

Of the many sources of information contributing to the production of this book, a few merit special mention:

The University of California, Los Angeles, deserves thanks and gratitude from problem sleepers everywhere, for their *NAPS* and *BEDS* online information programs. These invaluable services for the associated medical professions provide abstracts and links to both current developments and seminal works of research on the subject of sleep.

A far different (but no less important) resource is the *Library of the Future*®. This electronic compilation, a *World Library Product*®, was invaluable in locating material used in the preparation of the Sleep Book.

—J.G-G.

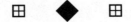

223

*Nothing is easier,
if a man wants it,
than rest.*
Henry Brooks Adams
The Education of Henry Adams, 1907.